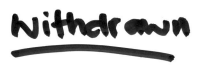

Contents

D11103593

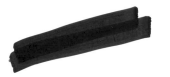

Contributors

Peter Boyle
Director of Division of Epidemiology and Biostatistics, European Institute, Milan, and Honorary Professor of Cancer Epidemiology, University of Birmingham

G A Chung-Faye
Clinical Research Fellow, Institute for Cancer Studies, University of Birmingham

T R P Cole
Consultant in Clinical Cancer Genetics, Birmingham Women's Hospital, Birmingham

Robert G Hardy
Wellcome Trust Clinical Research Fellow, Departments of Medicine and Surgery, University Hospital, Birmingham

F D Richard Hobbs
Professor, Department of Primary Care and General Practice, University of Birmingham

Janusz A Jankowski
Reader and Consultant Gastroenterologist, Department of Medicine, University Hospital, Birmingham and Imperial Cancer Research Fund, London

D J Kerr
Professor, Institute for Cancer Studies, University of Birmingham

Michael J S Langman
Professor of Medicine, University of Birmingham

Colin McArdle
Professor, University Department of Surgery, Royal Infirmary, Edinburgh

Stephen J Meltzer
Professor of Medicine and Director, Functional Genomics Laboratory, University of Maryland Greenbarn Cancer Centre, Baltimore, USA

Rachel S J Midgley
Clinical Research Fellow, CRC Institute for Cancer Studies, University of Birmingham

Daniel Rea
Senior Lecturer in Medical Oncology, Institute for Cancer Studies, University of Birmingham

John H Scholefield
Professor of Surgery, Division of Gastrointestinal Surgery, University Hospital, Nottingham

H V Sleightholme
Regional Cancer Coordinator, Department of Clinical Genetics, Birmingham Women's Hospital, Birmingham

Annie M Young
Research Fellow, School of Health Sciences, University of Birmingham

Preface

The inspiration for this book stemmed from the widely shared optimism of colorectal cancer specialists that after many decades of often painfully slow progress (despite much action), we are at the brink of a new era with several positive developments in the prevention, diagnosis and treatment of colorectal cancer, bringing hope to the hundreds of thousands of people who develop the disease.

It is crucial that this evidence-based sanguinity spreads to the entire multiprofessional colorectal cancer team, in particular to general practitioners who are by and large the first, the intermediate and the last point of contact for our patients. They have the complex task of firstly identifying suspected colorectal cancer and then working in partnership with the patient, carers and the specialists at all stages along the patient pathway. This book is written for them – the primary care physician, the nurses, the junior doctors, the dieticians, the radiographers and countless other healthcare professionals, all caring for colorectal cancer patients.

It isn't just that the book walks us through contemporary knowledge in the prevention, diagnosis, prognosis and modalities of treatment for colorectal cancer (and many other things besides) but it also acknowledges and debates the numerous uncertainties around the disease in a balanced manner, in addition to peering into future approaches towards screening, molecular biology, genetics and therapies.

The book, in short, presents a concise story of the full spectrum of colorectal cancer in a kind of chronological order. All of us who care for colorectal cancer patients, should make it our duty to be acquainted with the detail in order to provide optimal patient care.

Annie Young

1 Epidemiology

Peter Boyle, Michael J S Langman

In countries with a westernised lifestyle about half of all deaths are caused by circulatory disease and a quarter by cancer. Cancer is an important problem in both public health and political terms worldwide, irrespective of a country's development. The most recent estimates of the global cancer burden suggest that there were 8.1 million new cases, excluding non-melanoma skin cancer, worldwide in 1990. About 10 million new cases are now diagnosed each year.

Colorectal cancer is the fourth commonest form of cancer occurring worldwide, with an estimated 783 000 new cases diagnosed in 1990, the most recent year for which international estimates are available. It affects men and women almost equally, with about 401 000 new cases in men annually and 381 000 in women. The number of new cases of colorectal cancer worldwide has been increasing rapidly since 1975 (when it was 500 000).

Worldwide, colorectal cancer represents 9.4% of all incident cancer in men and 10.1% in women. Colorectal cancer, however, is not equally common throughout the world. If the westernised countries (North America; those in northern, southern, and western Europe; Australasia; and New Zealand) are combined, colorectal cancer represents 12.6% of all incident cancer in westernised countries in men and 14.1% in women. Elsewhere colorectal cancer represents 7.7% and 7.9% of all incident cases in men and women respectively.

Large differences exist in survival, according to the stage of disease. It is estimated that 394 000 deaths from colorectal cancer still occur worldwide annually, and colorectal cancer is the second commonest cause of death from any cancer in men in the European Union. Substantial differences in cancer survival seem to exist between Great Britain, Europe as a whole, and the United States. This variation in survival is not easily explained but could be related to stage of disease at presentation or treatment delivery, or both of these.

The numbers of new cases of colorectal cancer worldwide has increased rapidly since 1975

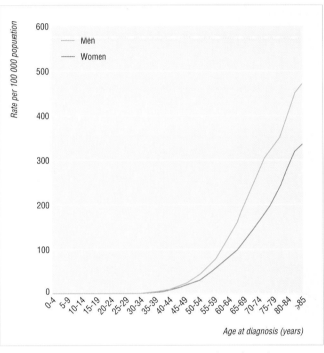

Figure 1.1 Estimated incidence of colorectal cancer in United Kingdom, by age and sex, 1995

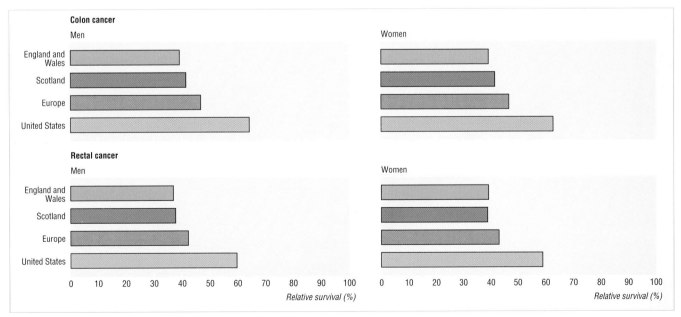

Figure 1.2 International comparison of five year relative survival for colon and rectal cancer in adults aged 15-99 at diagnosis (based on Coleman et al, *Cancer survival trends in England and Wales, 1971-1975*; Berrino et al, *Survival of cancer patients in Europe: the EUROCARE-2 study*; and Surveillance Epidemiology and End Results (SEER) programme, National Cancer Institute, 1998)

Survival and deprivation

The relation between poverty and ill health has been researched for more than 100 years. In Scotland, since the 1851 census, all cause occupational mortality has been routinely reported, and since 1911, inequalities in health, as shown by mortality, have been examined in decennial reports classified by social class (based on occupation) and by occupational group alone.

No single, generally agreed definition of deprivation exists. Deprivation is a concept that overlaps but is not synonymous with poverty. Absolute poverty can be defined as the absence of the minimum resources for physical survival, whereas relative poverty relates to the standards of living in a particular society. Deprivation includes material, social, and multiple deprivation. In Scotland the Carstairs and Morris index of deprivation was derived from 1981 census data with the postcode sector as the basic geographical unit (covering a population of about 5000). This index describes a deprivation category on a scale of 1 (least deprived) to 7 (most deprived) for each household address in Scotland.

The incidence of colorectal cancer is higher in men than women among each of the seven deprivation categories in Scotland, although incidence varies little with deprivation category. Survival, however, clearly improves with decreasing deprivation. At each milestone, there is a notable gradient in survival, with the most affluent doing best and the least affluent doing worst. The reasons that such variations exist are unclear and highlight an important priority for research.

Descriptive epidemiology

Different populations worldwide experience different levels of colorectal cancer, and these levels change with time. Populations living in one community whose lifestyles differ from those of others in the same community also experience different levels of colorectal cancer. Groups of migrants quickly lose the risk associated with their original home community and acquire the patterns of the new community, often starting within one generation of arrival.

Ethnic and racial differences in colorectal cancer, as well as studies on migrants, suggest that environmental factors play a major part in the aetiology of the disease. In Israel male Jews born in Europe or the United States are at higher risk of colon cancer than those born in Africa or Asia. Risk in the offspring of Japanese populations who have migrated to the United States has changed—incidence now approaches or surpasses that in white people in the same population and is three or four times higher than among the Japanese in Japan.

For reasons such as these, colorectal cancer is widely believed to be an environmental disease, with "environmental" defined broadly to include a wide range of ill defined cultural, social, and lifestyle practices. As much as 70-80% of colorectal cancers may owe their appearance to such factors; this clearly identifies colorectal cancer as one of the major neoplasms in which causes may be rapidly identified, and a large portion of the disease is theoretically avoidable.

The move from theoretically avoidable causes to implementation of preventive strategies depends on the identification of risk factors, exposures that have been associated with an increased (or decreased) risk of colorectal cancer, and the smaller subset of risk determinants, whose alteration would lead directly to a reduction in risk. From analytical epidemiology some clear ideas have now emerged about measures for reducing the risk of colorectal cancer.

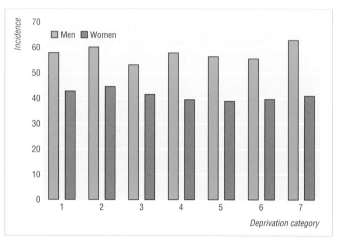

Figure 1.3 Incidence according to deprivation category in Scotland, 1998 (1=least deprived, 7=most deprived)

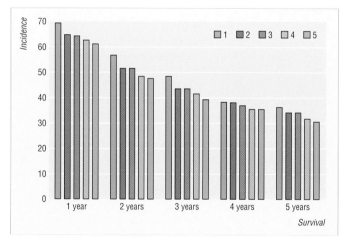

Figure 1.4 Survival according to deprivation category in Scotland, 1998 (1=least deprived, 5=most deprived)

Table 1.1 Highest incidence of colorectal cancer in men worldwide around 1990

Registry	Age standardised incidence per 100 000
US (Hawaii: Japanese), 1988-92	53.48
New Zealand (non-Maori), 1988-92	51.30
Japan (Hiroshima), 1986-90	50.99
France (Haut-Rhin), 1988-92	49.90
Italy (Trieste), 1989-92	49.37
France (Bas-Rhin), 1988-92	49.24
Canada (Yukon), 1983-92	48.98
US (Detroit: black), 1988-92	48.32
Czech Republic, 1988-92	48.23
US (Los Angeles: black), 1988-92	47.89
Canada (Nova Scotia), 1988-92	47.84
Canada (Newfoundland), 1988-92	47.29
Australia (New South Wales), 1988-92	46.92
US (San Francisco: black), 1988-92	46.82
Israel (Jews born in America or Europe), 1988-92	46.79

Data taken from Parkin et al, eds (*Cancer incidence in five continents*. Vol 7. IARC Scientific Publications, 1997:120)

Dietary and nutritional practices

Evidence from epidemiological studies seems to show consistently that intake of dietary fat and meat is positively related to risk of colorectal cancer. This evidence is obtained from ecological studies, animal experiments, and case-control and cohort studies.

In 1990 Willett et al published the results from the US nurses health study involving follow up of 88 751 women aged 34-59 years who were without cancer or inflammatory bowel disease at recruitment. After adjustment for total energy intake, consumption of animal fat was found to be associated with increased risk of colon cancer. The trend in risk was highly significant ($P = 0.01$), with the relative risk in the highest compared with the lowest quintile being 1.89 (95% confidence interval 1.13 to 3.15). No association was found with vegetable fat. The relative risk in women who ate beef, pork, or lamb as a main dish every day was 2.49 (1.24 to 5.03) compared with women reporting consumption less than once a month. The authors suggested that their data supported the hypothesis that a high intake of animal fat increases the risk of colon cancer, and they supported existing recommendations to substitute fish and chicken for meats high in fat.

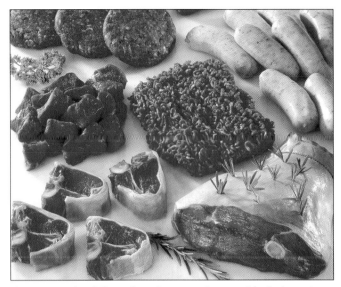

Figure 1.5 Intake of dietary fat and meat may increase risk of colorectal cancer

Intake of vegetables, fruit, and fibre

Dietary fibre has been proposed as accounting for the differences in the rates of colorectal cancer between Africa and westernised countries—on the basis that increased intake of dietary fibre may increase faecal bulk and reduce transit time. Various other factors, related to risk of colorectal cancer, are now thought to contribute to explaining these differences.

Fibre has many components, each of which has specific physiological functions. The components are most commonly grouped into insoluble, non-degradable constituents (mainly found in cereal fibre) and soluble, degradable constituents, such as pectin and plant gums (mainly found in fruits and vegetables). Epidemiological studies have reported differences in the effect of these components. Many studies, however, found no protective effect of fibre in cereals but have consistently found a protective effect of fibre in vegetables and perhaps fruits. This might reflect an association with other components of fruits and vegetables, with fibre intake acting merely as an indicator of consumption.

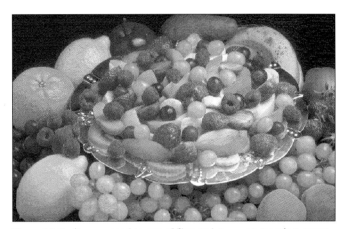

Figure 1.6 Fruits are a good source of fibre and may protect against cancer

Physical activity, body mass index, and energy intake

Evidence from epidemiological studies is strong that men with high occupational or recreational physical activity seem to have a decreased risk of colon cancer. Such evidence comes from follow up studies of cohorts who are physically active or who have physically demanding jobs, as well as from case-control studies that have assessed physical activity by, for example, measurement of resting heart rate or questionnaire. The association remains even after potential confounding factors, such as diet and body mass index, are controlled for.

The available data, however, show no consistent association between obesity and risk of colorectal cancer (analysis and interpretation of this factor is difficult in retrospective studies, where weight loss may be a sign of the disease), although evidence now suggests an association between obesity and adenomas. This increased risk associated with energy intake does not seem to be the result merely of overeating; it may reflect differences in metabolic efficiency. If the possibility that the association with energy intake is a methodological artefact is excluded (as such a consistent finding is unlikely to emerge from such a variety of study designs in diverse population groups), it would imply that individuals who use energy more efficiently may be at a lower risk of colorectal cancer.

Box 1.1 Physical activity and colorectal cancer

- Giovannucci et al examined the role of physical activity, body mass index, and the pattern of adipose distribution in the risk of colorectal adenomas
- In the nurses health study, 13 057 female nurses, aged 40-65 years in 1986, had an endoscopy during 1986-92. During this period, adenoma of the distal colorectum was newly diagnosed in 439 nurses
- After age, prior endoscopy, parental history of colorectal cancer, smoking, aspirin use, and dietary intake were controlled for, physical activity was associated inversely with the risk of large adenomas (≥ 1 cm) in the distal colon (relative risk 0.57 (95% confidence interval 0.30 to 1.08)) when high and low quintiles of average weekly energy expenditure from leisure activities were compared
- Much of this benefit came from activities of moderate intensity, such as brisk walking

---

Hormone replacement therapy

Increasing evidence supports an (originally unexpected) association between hormone replacement therapy and a reduced risk of colorectal cancer.

Of 19 published studies of hormonal replacement therapy and risk of colorectal cancer, 10 support an inverse association and a further five show a significant reduction in risk. The risk seems lowest among long term users. Although some contradictions still exist in the available literature, hormone replacement therapy seems likely to reduce the risk of colorectal cancer in women. The risk seems to halve with 5-10 years' use. The role of unopposed versus combination hormone replacement therapy needs further research.

Whether this association is causal or is associated with some selection factor that directs women to using hormone replacement therapy is, however, not known. This question is important; if the link is indeed causal, women who are at high risk of colorectal cancer could be offered the therapy to lower their risk.

Control of colorectal cancer

Prospects for preventing death from colorectal cancer are now more promising than even 10 years ago. To achieve this goal public health decisions have to be taken, and part of this decision process involves deciding at which point enough epidemiological evidence is available to change focus comfortably from information generation to health actions.

To turn research findings into public health strategies for controlling the incidence of and mortality from colorectal cancer requires a profound change of mentality in the epidemiological community. It is easy to say that more studies are needed, but they would be unlikely to alter existing conclusions. Moreover, the implementation of strategies to control cancer must be considered separately from research into the control of cancer.

One consequence of epidemiological research into the contribution of lifestyle factors to cancer risk has been to blame the individual who develops cancer. Smoking, alcohol, dietary imprudence, and exposure to sunlight tend to assign responsibility to the individual. The individual is often not principally responsible for decisions about factors that influence his or her risk of cancer, and society—including government and industry—could do more to discourage lifestyles associated with cancer risk. Government legislation, including taxation policy and other actions, could have profound effects on smoking habits, for example.

The goal of all cancer research and treatment is to prevent people dying from the disease. Knowledge has been accruing rapidly about actions and interventions that could lead to a reduction in death from colorectal cancer by reducing the risk of developing the disease, identifying the disease at a stage when it is more curable, or improving the outcome of treatment.

Box 1.2 How individuals can reduce their risk of colorectal cancer

- Increase intake of vegetables and fruits (eat five servings of fruits and vegetables each day); replace snacks such as chocolate, biscuits, and crisps with an apple, orange, or other fruit or vegetable
- Reduce intake of calories (animal fats in particular); often replace beef, lamb, and pork with fish and poultry
- Increase physical activity—by activities of moderate intensity, such as brisk walking
- Participate in population screening programmes; when these are not in place, strongly consider having a colonoscopy with polyp removal once between ages 50 and 59
- Consult a doctor as soon as possible if a noticeable and unexplained change in bowel habits occurs, blood is present in the stool, colicky pain occurs in the abdomen, or a sensation of incomplete evacuation after defecation recurs

---

Further reading

- Boyle P. Progress in preventing death from colorectal cancer [editorial]. *Br J Cancer* 1995;72:528-30.
- Berrino F, Capocaccia R, Estève J, Gatta G, Hakulinen T, Micheli A, et al, eds. *Survival of cancer patients in Europe: the EUROCARE-2 study.* Lyons: International Agency for Research on Cancer, 1999. (Scientific publication No 151.)
- Coleman MP, Babb P, Damiecki P, Grosclaude P, Honjo S, Jones J, et al. Cancer survival trends in England and Wales, 1971-1995: deprivation and NHS region. London: Stationery Office, 1999.
- Giovannucci E, Colditz GA, Stampfer MJ, Willett WC. Physical activity, obesity and risk of colorectal cancer in women (United States). *Cancer Causes Control* 1996;7:253-63.
- McLaren G, Bain M. *Deprivation and health in Scotland: insights from NHS data.* Edinburgh: ISD Scotland, 1998.
- MacLennan SC, MacLennan AH, Ryan P. Colorectal cancer and oestrogen replacement therapy: a meta-analysis of epidemiological studies. *Med J Aust* 1991;162:491-3.
- Parkin DM, Pisani P, Ferlay J. Estimates of the worldwide incidence of 25 major cancers in 1990. *Int J Cancer* 1999;80:827-41.
- Shephard RJ. Exercise in the prevention and treatment of cancer—an update. *Sports Med* 1993;15:258-80.
- Willett WC. The search for the causes of breast and colon cancer. *Nature* 1989;338:389-94.
- Willett WC, Stampfer MJ, Colditz GA, Rosner BA, Speizer FE. Relation of meat, fat, and fiber intake to the risk of colon cancer in a prospective study among women. *N Engl J Med* 1990;323:1664-72.

The two graphs showing incidence of colorectal cancer in the United Kingdom and an international comparison of five year relative survival for colon and rectal cancer are adapted with permission from the Cancer Research Campaign (*CRC CancerStats: Large Bowel—UK*; factsheet, November 1999) The graphs of incidence and survival according to deprivation category are adapted from McLaren G et al (*Deprivation and health in Scotland.* ISD Scotland Publications, 1998). The photograph of meat is published with permission from Tim Hall/CEPHAS.

2 Molecular basis for risk factors

Robert G Hardy, Stephen J Meltzer, Janusz A Jankowski

Evidence for the molecular basis of colorectal cancer comes from genetic analysis of tissues either from patients with a family history of the disease or from patients with sporadic adenomatous colorectal polyps or extensive ulcerative colitis. The traditional view is that background rates of genetic mutation, combined with several rounds of clonal expansion, are necessary for a tumour to develop. It has recently been argued, however, that inherent genetic instability not only is necessary but may also be sufficient for cancer to develop.

Sporadic colorectal adenomas

More than 70% of colorectal cancers develop from sporadic adenomatous polyps, and postmortem studies have shown the incidence of adenomas to be 30-40% in Western populations. Polyps are asymptomatic in most cases and are often multiple. Flat adenomas, which are more difficult to detect at endoscopy, account for about 10% of all polyps and may have a higher rate of malignant change or may predispose to a more aggressive cancer phenotype.

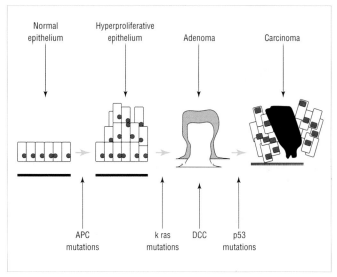

Figure 2.1 Proposed adenoma to carcinoma sequence in colorectal cancer. Adenomatous polyposis coli (APC) gene mutations and hypermethylation occur early, followed by k ras mutations. Deleted in colon cancer (DCC) and p53 gene mutations occur later in the sequence, although the exact order may vary

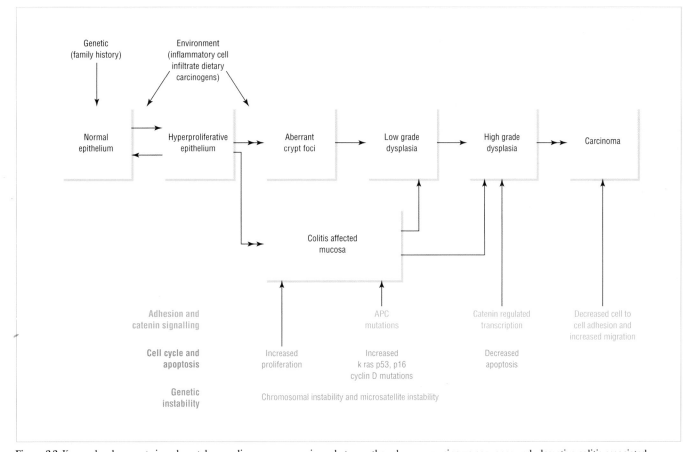

Figure 2.2 Key molecular events in colorectal premalignancy: comparisons between the adenoma carcinoma sequence and ulcerative colitis associated neoplasia

Family history

Recognised familial syndromes account for about 5% of colorectal cancers. The commonest hereditary syndromes are familial adenomatous polyposis and heredity non-polyposis colon cancer. Patients with these syndromes usually have a family history of colorectal cancer presenting at an early age. Attenuated familial adenomatous polyposis, juvenile polyposis syndrome, and Peutz-Jeghers syndrome are rarer, mendelian causes of colorectal cancer. In familial adenomatous polyposis (a mendelian dominant disorder with almost complete penetrance) there is a germline mutation in the tumour suppressor gene for adenomatous polyposis coli (APC) on chromosome 5.

Heredity non-polyposis colon cancer also shows dominant inheritance, and cancers develop mainly in the proximal colon. Patients with heredity non-polyposis colon cancer show germline mutations in DNA mismatch repair enzymes (which normally remove misincorporated single or multiple nucleotide bases as a result of random errors during recombination or replications). Mutations are particularly demonstrable in DNA with multiple microsatellites ("microsatellite instability").

In addition to the well recognised syndromes described above, clusters of colorectal cancer occur in families much more often than would be expected by chance. Postulated reasons for this increased risk include "mild" APC and mismatch repair gene mutations, as well as polymorphisms of genes involved in nutrient or carcinogen metabolism.

Box 2.1 Factors determining risk of malignant transformation within colonic adenomatous polyps

High risk
Large size (especially > 1.5 cm)
Sessile or flat
Severe dysplasia
Presence of squamous metaplasia
Villous architecture
Polyposis syndrome (multiple polyps)

Low risk
Small size (especially < 1.0 cm)
Pedunculated
Mild dysplasia
No metaplastic areas
Tubular architecture
Single polyp

The immediate family members of a patient with colorectal cancer will have a twofold to threefold increased risk of the disease

---

Table 2.1 Clinical and molecular correlates of familial adenomatous polyposis coli; attenuated familial adenomatous polyposis coli/hereditary flat adenoma syndrome; hereditary non-polyposis colon cancer/Lynch forms of hereditary colorectal cancer; and ulcerative colitis associated neoplasia

	FAP	AFAP/HFAS	HNPCC/Lynch	UCAN
Mean age at diagnosis of colorectal cancer	32-39	45-55	42-49	40-70
Distribution of cancer	Random	Mainly right colon	Mainly right colon	Mainly left colon
No of polyps	>100	1-100	1 (ie tumour)	
Sex ratio (male:female)	1:1	1:1	1.5:1	1:1
Endoscopic view of polyp	Pedunculated	Mainly flat	Pedunculated (45%); flat (55%)	None
Lag time (years) from early adenoma to occurrence of cancer	10-20	10	5	$?<8$
Proportion (%) of colonic cancer	1	0.5	1-5	<0.5
Superficial physical stigmata	80% have retinal pigmentation	None	Only in Muir-Torre syndrome	None
Distribution of polyps	Distal colon or universal	Mainly proximal to splenic flexure with rectal sparing	Mainly proximal to splenic flexure	None
Carcinoma histology	More exophytic growth	Non-exophytic but very variable	Inflammation increased mucin	Mucosal ulceration and inflammation
Other associated tumours	Duodenal adenoma cerebral and thyroid tumours, medulloblastoma and desmoids	Duodenal adenoma	Endometrial ovarian, gastric cancer, glioblastoma, many other cancers	
Gene (chromosome) mutation	APC (5q 21) distal to 5′	APC (5q 21) proximal to 5′	MHS2 (2p), MLH1 (3p21), PMS1 (2q31), PMS2 (7p22)	Multiple mutations, 17p (p53), 5q (APC), 9p (p16)

FAP = familial adenomatous polyposis coli; AFAP = attenuated familial adenomatous polyposis coli; HFAS = hereditary flat adenoma syndrome; HNPPC = hereditary non-polyposis colon cancer; UCAN = ulcerative colitis associated neoplasia.

Risk from ulcerative colitis

Several studies have indicated that patients with ulcerative colitis have a 2-8.2 relative risk of colorectal cancer compared with the normal population, accounting for about 2% of colorectal cancers. One of the factors influencing an individual's risk is duration of colitis—the cumulative incidence of colorectal cancer is 5% at 15 years and 8-13% at 25 years. The extent of disease is also important: patients with involvement of right and transverse colon are more likely to develop colorectal cancer (the relative risk in these patients is 15 compared with the normal population). Coexisting primary sclerosing cholangitis independently increases the relative risk of ulcerative colitis associated neoplasia (UCAN) by 3-15%. In addition, high grade dysplasia in random rectosigmoid biopsies is associated with an unsuspected cancer at colectomy in 33% of patients.

Molecular basis of adenoma carcinoma sequence and UCAN

Cancers arising in colitis versus those in adenomas

Important clinical and biological differences exist between the adenoma carcinoma sequence and ulcerative colitis associated neoplasia. Firstly, cancer in ulcerative colitis probably evolves from microscopic dysplasia with or without a mass lesion rather than from adenomas. Secondly, the time interval from the presence of adenoma to progression to carcinoma probably exceeds the interval separating ulcerative colitis associated dysplasia from ulcerative colitis associated neoplasia. Thirdly, patients with a family history of colorectal cancer (but not ulcerative colitis associated neoplasia) and who also have ulcerative colitis are at further increased risk, suggesting additive factors.

Chromosomal instability

Aneuploidy indicates gross losses or gains in chromosomal DNA and is often seen in many human primary tumours and premalignant conditions. It has been shown that aneuploid "fields" tend to populate the epithelium of patients with ulcerative colitis even in histologically benign colitis. These changes may occur initially in some cases by loss of one allele at a chromosomal locus (loss of heterozygosity) and may imply the presence of a tumour suppressor gene at that site. Loss of both alleles at a given locus (homozygous deletion) is an even stronger indicator of the existence of a tumour suppressor gene. Loss of heterozygosity occurs clonally in both the adenoma carcinoma sequence and ulcerative colitis associated neoplasia. Many of these loci are already associated with one or more known candidate tumour suppressor genes. These include 3p21 (β catenin gene), 5q21 (APC gene), 9p (p16 and p15 genes), 13q (retinoblastoma gene), 17p (p53 gene), 17q (BRCA1 gene), 18q (DCC and SMAD4 genes), and less frequently 16q (E cadherin gene).

The p53 gene locus is the commonest site demonstrating loss of heterozygosity. p53 is a DNA binding protein transcriptional activator and can arrest the cell cycle in response to DNA damage—hence its title "guardian of the genome." The effect of normal (wild-type) p53 is antagonised by mutation or by action of the antiapoptotic gene Bcl-2, which is significantly less frequently overexpressed in ulcerative colitis associated neoplasia than in the adenoma carcinoma sequence. Most mutations in p53 cause the protein to become hyperstable and lead to its accumulation in the nucleus.

A second tumour suppressor gene necessary for development of sporadic colorectal cancer is APC, which is

---

Box 2.2 Factors affecting risk of colorectal cancer in patients with ulcerative colitis

High risk
Long duration of disease (especially > 10 years)
Extensive disease
Dysplasia
Presence of primary sclerosing cholangitis
Family history of colorectal cancer
Coexisting adenomatous polyp

Low risk
Short duration of disease (especially < 10 years)
Proctitis only
No dysplasia
No primary sclerosing cholangitis
No family history of colorectal cancer
No coexisting adenomatous polyp

Box 2.3 Chromosomal and microsatellite instability

- Molecular alterations in colorectal cancer can be grouped into two broad categories: chromosomal instability (subdivided into aneuploidy and chromosomal alterations) and microsatellite instability
- As a consequence of these two phenomena, other specific genetic events occur at increased frequency
- These include inactivation of tumour suppressor genes by deletion or mutation, activation of proto-oncogenes by mutation, and dysregulated expression of diverse molecules, such as the cell to cell adhesion molecule E cadherin and mucin related sialosyl-Tn antigen

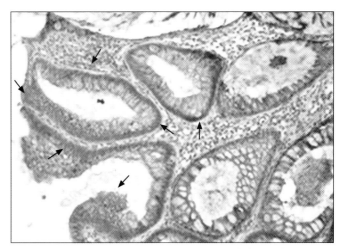

Figure 2.3 Downregulation of E cadherin (arrowed) within colonic adenoma. Normal membranous E cadherin staining (brown) is seen in non-dysplastic crypts in the right of the picture

inactivated in >80% of early colorectal cancers. Consequently this gene has been termed the "gatekeeper" for adenoma development as adenoma formation requires perturbation of the APC gene's function or that of related proteins such as catenins. An important function of the APC gene is to prevent the accumulation of molecules associated with cancer, such as catenins. Accumulation of catenins can lead to the transcription of the oncogene c-myc, giving a proliferative advantage to the cell. APC mutations occur later and are somewhat less common in ulcerative colitis associated neoplasia (4-27%) than in sporadic colorectal adenomas and carcinomas. Catenins also bind E cadherin, which functions as a tumour suppressor gene in the gastrointestinal tract. It is currently thought that mutated catenins may not bind to APC and thus accumulate.

Microsatellite instability

A further important category of alteration studied in the adenoma carcinoma sequence and ulcerative colitis associated neoplasia is microsatellite instability. This comprises length alterations of oligonucleotide repeat sequences that occur somatically in human tumours. This mechanism is also responsible for the germline defects found in heredity non-polyposis colon cancer. The incidence of microsatellite instability has been noted to be about 15% for adenomas and 25% for colorectal cancers overall. Microsatellite instability also occurs in patients with ulcerative colitis and is fairly common in premalignant (dysplastic) and malignant lesions (21% and 19% respectively). Indeed it has also been reported in "histologically normal" ulcerative colitis mucosa. It can therefore be considered to be an early event in the adenoma carcinoma sequence and in ulcerative colitis associated neoplasia.

Prognosis

The prognosis of colorectal cancer is determined by both pathological and molecular characteristics of the tumour.

Pathology

Pathology has an essential role in the staging of colorectal cancer. There has been a gradual move from using Dukes's classification to using the TNM classification system as this is thought to lead to a more accurate, independent description of the primary tumour and its spread. More advanced disease naturally leads to reduced disease-free interval and survival. Independent factors affecting survival include incomplete resection margins, grade of tumour, and number of lymph nodes involved (particularly apical node metastasis—main node draining a lymphatic segment).

Molecular biology

Reports on correlations between tumour genotype and prognosis are currently incomplete. However, analysis of survival data from patients with sporadic colorectal cancer and from those with colorectal cancer associated with familial adenomatous polyposis and hereditary non-polyposis colon cancer has not shown any reproducible significant differences between these groups. In premalignancy, however, the onset of p53 mutations in histologically normal mucosa in ulcerative colitis suggests that detection of such mutations may be a useful strategy in determining mucosal areas with a high risk of dysplastic transformation.

E cadherin mutations are not commonly associated with the adenoma carcinoma sequence, but loss of heterozygosity and, rarely, missense mutations have been reported in 5% of ulcerative colitis associated neoplasia

Table 2.2 Staging and survival of colorectal cancers

TNM classification	Modified Dukes's classification	Survival (%)
Stage 0—Carcinoma in situ		
Stage I—No nodal involvement, no metastases; tumour invades submucosa (T1, N0, M0); tumour invades muscularis propria (T2, N0, M0)	A	90-100
Stage II—No nodal involvement, no metastases; tumour invades into subserosa (T3, N0, M0); tumour invades other organs (T4, N0, M0)	B	75-85
Stage III—Regional lymph nodes involved (any T, N1, M0)	C	30-40
Stage IV—Distant metastases	D	<5

Further reading

- Oates GD, Finan PJ, Marks CG, Bartram CI, Reznek RH, Shepherd NA, et al. *Handbook for the clinico-pathological assessment and staging of colorectal cancer.* London: UK Co-ordinating Committee on Cancer Research, 1997.
- Lengauer C, Kinzler KW, Vogelstein B. Genetic instabilities in human cancers. *Nature* 1998;396:643-9.
- Tomlinson I, Bodmer W. Selection, the mutation rate and cancer: ensuring that the tail does not wag the dog. *Nature Med* 1999;5:11-2.
- Powell SM, Zilz N, Beazer-Barclay Y, Bryan TM, Hamilton SR, Thibodeau SN, et al. APC mutations occur early during colorectal tumorigenesis. *Nature* 1992;359:235-7.
- Jankowski J, Bedford F, Boulton RA, Cruickshank N, Hall C, Elder J, et al. Alterations in classical cadherins in the progression of ulcerative and Crohn's colitis. *Lab Invest* 1998;78:1155-67.
- Fearon ER, Vogelstein B. A genetic model for colorectal tumorigenesis. *Cell* 1990;61:759-67.
- Liu B, Parsons R, Papadopoulos N, Nicolaides NC, Lynch HT, Watson P, et al. Analysis of mismatch repair genes in hereditary non-polyposis colorectal cancer patients. *Nature Med* 1996;2:169-74.

This work was funded by the Cancer Research Campaign and the Medical Research Department of Veteran Affairs. Fiona K Bedford, Robert Allan, Michael Langman, William Doe, and Dion Morton provided useful comments.

3   The role of clinical genetics in management

T R P Cole, H V Sleightholme

Before 1990 the role of inherited factors in the aetiology of adult cancer was relatively poorly understood and aroused little interest among doctors and the public alike—although familial adenomatous polyposis (the autosomal dominant colon cancer syndrome) was an exception in this respect. In the past decade, however, interest has increased markedly. In the West Midlands, for example, familial cancer referrals constituted < 1% (< 20 cases) of all clinical genetic referrals in 1991, whereas now they represent over 30% of cases (> 1000).

Despite the estimate that 5-10% of colorectal cancer has an inherited basis, only a small percentage of referred families have mutations in one of the currently identified genes. Furthermore, mutation studies are usually possible only if DNA is available from an affected patient, so molecular investigation will facilitate the management of only a small minority of cases. The remaining referrals must be managed with clinically derived strategies. This article discusses the clinical features and management of dominant colon cancer syndromes and provides referral guidelines and screening protocols for more common familial clusters.

Genetic counselling for families with a history of cancer requires a full and accurate family history. When possible, histological confirmation of the reported tumours should be obtained. It should then be possible to recognise the specific cancer syndromes. It is important to emphasise to families that however extensive the family history of cancer (unless present on both sides), a person will always have a greater than 50% chance of not developing that particular tumour. This may surprise but greatly reassure many families.

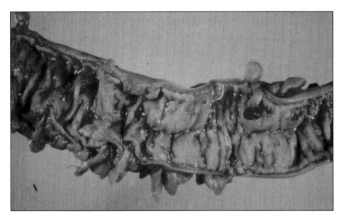

Figure 3.1 Number of referrals of patients with cancer (except familial adenomatous polyposis) to West Midlands regional clinical genetics service, 1988-98

Familial adenomatous polyposis

Familial adenomatous polyposis, previously called polyposis coli (or Gardner's syndrome if extra colonic manifestations were present), is the best recognised of the colorectal cancer syndromes but accounts for less than 1% of all colorectal cancers and has an incidence of 1 in 10 000. It is characterised by the presence of 100 or more tubovillous adenomas in the colon, with intervening microadenoma on histological examination. The mean age of diagnosis of polyps is during teenage years, and almost all of gene carriers have polyps by the age of 40. If these polyps are left untreated, malignant transformation is inevitable, with a mean age of colorectal cancer occurring during the patients' mid-30s, often with synchronous tumours.

This condition is an autosomal dominant disorder, with the offspring of affected individuals at 50% risk of being gene carriers. The diagnosis of familial adenomatous polyposis should always result in a careful and full evaluation of the family history. Wherever possible, parents should have at least one colonoscopy, irrespective of age. In most cases without a family history, parental examination will be negative and the proband will probably be one of 30% of cases that represent new mutations. The siblings of all probands, however, should be offered annual flexible sigmoidoscopy up to the age of 40 or until proved to be non-gene carriers.

The cloning of the causative gene (APC) on chromosome 5 in 1991 dramatically changed the management of familial adenomatous polyposis. If DNA is available from an affected

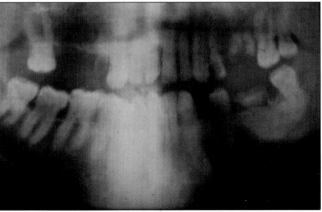

Figure 3.2 Features of familial adenomatous polyposis: colon with multiple polyps (top) and jaw cysts (bottom)

individual, mutation detection is possible in about 70% of families. In these families first degree relatives should be offered predictive testing with appropriate genetic counselling. In families with no identified mutation, linkage studies to identify the "high risk" chromosome 5 are possible in many cases. Non-gene carriers should be reassured and surveillance stopped. Gene carriers should be offered annual flexible sigmoidoscopy from the age of 12. Once several polyps have been identified, the timing and type of surgery available should be discussed (a sensitive issue in teenagers and young adults). The two most common options are ileal-rectal anastomosis with annual surveillance of the remaining rectal tissue; and ileal-anal anastomosis with reconstruction of a rectal pouch using terminal small bowel.

Molecular testing is usually offered to "at risk" children at age 10-14 before starting annual sigmoidoscopy. However, parental pressure for earlier testing (before the child can give consent) is not uncommon, and ongoing studies may help to clarify when to proceed with testing.

Cloning APC explained several clinical features and aided studies of genotypes and phenotypes. For example, congenital hypertrophy of the retinal pigment epithelium, an attenuated phenotype (that is, fewer than 100 polyps or late onset), and non-malignant but debilitating and potentially lethal desmoid disease each show an association with mutations in specific exon regions. The cloning also confirmed clinical findings that familial adenomatous polyposis and Gardner's syndrome were different manifestations of the same disease spectrum that could coexist within the same family.

With greater clinical awareness, regular surveillance, and the advent of molecular investigation, almost all colorectal cancer deaths in inherited cases of familial adenomatous polyposis can be avoided. Increased survival has revealed later complications, in particular periampullary or duodenal adenocarcinoma (present in about 12% of postcolectomy cases). Also important are aggressive desmoid disease and other rare malignant disease.

Chemoprophylactic approaches to reduce polyp growth (for example, aspirin and non-digestible starch) are the subject of multicentre trials.

Hereditary non-polyposis colon cancer

Hereditary non-polyposis colon cancer (also known as Lynch syndrome) became more widely recognised about 30 years ago in families manifesting mainly colorectal cancer segregating in an autosomal dominant fashion. Many families also exhibit extracolonic tumours, particularly gynaecological, small bowel, or urinary tract carcinomas, and these became known as Lynch type 2 to distinguish them from site specific colorectal cancers, designated Lynch type 1. The subsequent name change to hereditary non-polyposis colon cancer is potentially misleading as many gene carriers will develop a small number of tubovillous adenomas, but not more than 100, as seen in familial adenomatous polyposis. The proportion of colorectal cancers due to hereditary non-polyposis colon cancer is controversial, and estimates range from 1% to 20%; most observers, however, suggest about 2%.

The diagnosis of hereditary non-polyposis colon cancer is made on the family history as the appearance of the bowel, unlike in familial adenomatous polyposis, is not diagnostic. To improve the recognition of hereditary non-polyposis colon cancer, diagnostic criteria were devised in Amsterdam in 1991 and were subsequently modified to include non-colonic tumours.

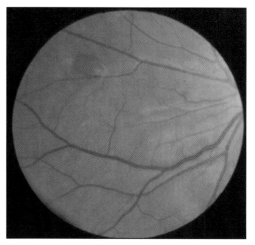

Figure 3.3 Congenital hypertrophy of the retinal pigmentary epithelium is a feature of familial adenomatous polyposis

---

Box 3.1 Early and late extracolonic tumours in familial adenomatous polyposis

- Hepatoblastoma (early)
- Adrenal adenoma (early or late)
- Desmoid disease (early or late)
- Papillary thyroid cancer—females only (late)
- Periampullary carcinoma (late)

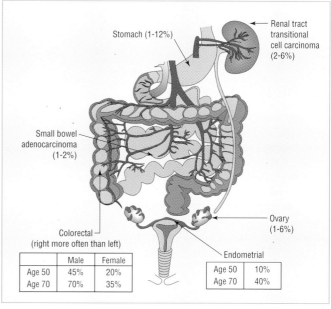

Figure 3.4 Site of tumours and frequency in hereditary non-polyposis colon cancer (upper figures in ranges may be overestimates owing to ascertainment bias)

Box 3.2 Modified Amsterdam criteria

- Three or more cases of colorectal cancer in a minimum of two generations
- One affected individual must be a first degree relative of the other two (or more) cases
- One case must be diagnosed before age 50
- Colorectal cancer can be replaced by endometrial or small bowel adenocarcinoma
- Familial adenomatous polyposis must be excluded

In 1994 the first of the genes for hereditary non-polyposis colon cancer (hMSH2 on chromosome 2) was cloned, and since then four further genes have been identified; all are mismatch repair genes. If both copies of the genes are mutated, as postulated in Knudson's "two hit" hypothesis, that cell and all its daughter cells are missing a vital mechanism for repair of DNA in somatic tissue. Failure to repair mutations in tumour suppressor genes will in some instances result in initiation of the adenoma carcinoma sequence. Molecular studies showed that about 30% of colorectal cancers with early onset (under age 35) are due to the mismatch repair genes, and the typical age of onset and the spectrum of tumours in families with hereditary non-polyposis colon cancer were revised.

The limited available evidence suggests that screening for colorectal cancer in hereditary non-polyposis colon cancer is beneficial. In 1999 Vasen et al published figures showing clinical benefit and cost effectiveness of screening in hereditary non-polyposis colon cancer after a Finnish study reporting reduced morbidity and mortality in a non-randomised observational study of colonoscopy versus no screening.

The optimal surveillance frequency has not yet been defined in families with hereditary non-polyposis colon cancer. The method of choice, however, is colonoscopy rather than flexible sigmoidoscopy as 80% of cancers are proximal to the rectum (compared with only 57% in sporadic colorectal cancer). The screening interval should be at most three years and probably every 18-24 months in gene carriers. Failure to reach the caecum should be followed by barium enema examination, although surveillance using radiological techniques should probably be used sparingly owing to the theoretical mutagenic consequences in patients with DNA repair defects. Patients should understand that the strategy of colonoscopy is the removal of polyps and prevention of tumours or early diagnosis, but that complete prevention is impossible.

Familial clusters with no recognisable single gene disorder

Families whose cancers do not meet the diagnostic criteria of familial adenomatous polyposis, hereditary non-polyposis colon cancer, or rarer colorectal cancer syndromes (such as syndromes related to the PTEN gene, Turcot's syndrome, Peutz-Jeghers syndrome, or juvenile polyposis) make up the largest and most difficult group of patients requesting management. There is rarely any indication of the aetiological basis of the cluster of colorectal cancer, and many instances will be coincidental occurrences. Other tumours clusters may be due to common environmental exposures, the effect of multiple low penetrance genes, or an interaction of both these elements. The risk of colorectal cancer may be assessed with empirical risk figures. These figures are estimates, however, and do not take into account factors such as the number of unaffected relatives. Further enquiry is usually justified if features such as multiple relatives with the same tumour or early onset of tumours are present in a family.

Concerns about not having precise risk figures may be misguided as many patients have difficulty interpreting risk figures and are often requesting only general guidance on risk and a discussion of management options. Many different screening protocols have been suggested in the past, however, and the lack of consistency and long term audit in these families is a problem.

To manage familial cancer in the West Midlands (population 5.2 million), a protocol has been developed that builds on the Calman-Hine model for cancer services and maximise the role

No large series of patients fulfilling the Amsterdam criteria has a mutation detection rate >70%. The figure is much lower for families that do not meet the criteria described here. Case selection using tumour DNA instability or immunohistochemical studies can improve mutation detection rates

- **Screening of other organ systems has not yet been proved beneficial**
- **It is prudent to screen for gynaecological tumours in mutation positive families, irrespective of family history, as 40% of female gene carriers develop endometrial carcinomas**
- **If tumours have been identified in the gynaecological or urinary tract in the family, surveillance should be offered (see the West Midlands guidelines)**

Box 3.3 West Midlands site specific screening strategies in hereditary non-polyposis colon cancer

Colorectal (all cases)—colonoscopy every two years at age 25-65
Endometrial*—annual pipelle biopsy (suction curettage) and ultrasound at age 30-65
Ovarian†—annual transvaginal ultrasound and serum Ca125 concentration at age 30-65
Transitional cell carcinoma in the urinary tract—annual haematuria test at age 25-40; annual urine cytology at age 40-65 (with or without cystoscopy every one to two years); annual renal ultrasound at age 40-65

*Families with history of endometrial cancer and mutation positive families.
†Families with history of ovarian cancer.

Table 3.1 Lifetime risk of colorectal cancer in first degree relatives of patient with colorectal cancer (from Houlston et al, 1990)

Population risk	1 in 50
One first degree relative affected (any age)	1 in 17
One first degree and one second degree relative affected	1 in 12
One first degree relative affected (age <45)	1 in 10
Two first degree relatives affected	1 in 6
Autosomal dominant pedigree	1 in 2

Box 3.4 Four pointers to recognition of familial cancer clusters

- High frequency of the same tumour in the family
- Early age of onset of tumours
- Multiple primary tumours
- Recognised associations—for example, colorectal and endometrial adenocarcinomas

of primary care. The protocol provides clear inclusion and screening guidance for cancer units and centres. This has promoted a consistency of management in and between families and is now allowing data collection for audit.

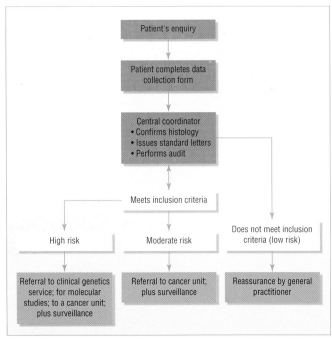

Figure 3.5 Algorithm for West Midlands family cancer strategy

It may be wise for general practitioners to use a reactive approach to patient enquiries until evidence exists to support a proactive approach. In the West Midlands, patients requesting advice are asked to complete a data collection sheet at home. This form and the inclusion criteria are available at www.bham.ac.uk/ich/clingen.htm. Completion of the form in the patient's own time, at home, facilitates discussion with relatives to clarify the relevant information and has saved time in primary care if a referral is required.

After histological confirmation in suspected familial cases, the data are evaluated centrally to identify high risk families requiring specialist investigation or referral to a cancer unit.

In a pilot study (population 200 000) the protocol reduced referrals from primary care by 50%, with a greater reduction in screening owing to a fall in low risk referrals to cancer units. This was associated with an increased referral rate for high risk referrals to clinical genetics departments. Central coordination prevents unnecessary investigations for different branches of any one family and facilitates audit.

Reports from general practitioners and patients suggest that individuals at no or minimal increased risk of cancer avoid unnecessary outpatient appointments and screening and for the most part are reassured by standardised protocols with explanations on the data collection forms. Such systems need to be studied further but seem to be preferable to continuing the current exponential rise of ad hoc responses from individual clinicians without long term audit.

Table 3.2 West Midlands inclusion and screening criteria for a family history of colorectal cancer

Inclusion criteria	Screening method	Age range (years) for surveillance
One first degree relative aged >40	Reassure, plus general advice on symptoms	Not applicable
One first degree relative aged <40	Colonoscopy every 5 years; appointment at local screening unit	25-65, or 5 years before tumour if later
Two first degree relatives average age >70	Reassure, plus general advice on symptoms	Not applicable
Two first degree relatives average age 60-70	Single colonoscopy; appointment at local screening unit	About 55
Two first degree relatives average age 50-60	Colonoscopy every 5 years; appointment at local screening unit	35-65
Two first degree relatives average age <50	Colonoscopy every 3-5 years; referral to genetics unit	30-65
Three close relatives but not meeting Amsterdam criteria	Colonoscopy every 3-5 years; referral to genetics unit	Begin age 30-40; stop at 65
Three close relatives meeting Amsterdam criteria	Colonoscopy every 2 years; referral to genetics unit	25-65
Familial adenomatous polyposis	Annual sigmoidoscopy; referral to genetics unit	12-40

Further reading

- Foulkes W. A tale of four syndromes: familial adenomatous polyposis, Gardner syndrome, attenuated APC and Turcot syndrome. *Q J Med* 1995;88:853-63.
- Vasen HF, van Ballegooijen, Buskens E, Kleibeuker JK, Taal BG, Griffioen G, et al. A cost-effectiveness analysis of colorectal screening of hereditary nonpolyposis colorectal carcinoma gene carriers. *Cancer* 1998;82:1632-7.
- Burke W, Petersen G, Lynch P, Bokin J, Daly M, Garber J, et al. Recommendations for follow-up care of individuals with an inherited predisposition to cancer. 1: Hereditary nonpolyposis colon cancer. *JAMA* 1997;277:915-9.
- Houlston RS, Murday V, Harocopos C, Williams CB, Slack J. Screening and genetic counselling for relatives of patients with colorectal cancer in a family cancer clinic. *BMJ* 1990;301:366-8.
- Hodgson SV, Maher ER, eds. *A practical guide to human cancer genetics*. Cambridge: Cambridge University Press, 1999.

Professor Eamonn Maher gave helpful comments and support.

4 Screening

John H Scholefield

Colorectal cancer is the third commonest malignancy in the United Kingdom, after lung and breast cancer, and kills about 20 000 people a year. It is equally prevalent in men and women, usually occurring in later life (at age 60-70 years). The incidence of the disease has generally increased over recent decades in both developed and developing countries. Despite this trend, mortality in both sexes has slowly declined. This decrease in mortality may reflect a trend towards earlier diagnosis—perhaps as a result of increased public awareness of the disease.

Surgery remains the mainstay of treatment for colorectal cancer, but early diagnosis makes it more likely that the tumour can be completely resected and thereby improves the chance of cure

Why screen?

Most colorectal cancers result from malignant change in polyps (adenomas) that have developed in the lining of the bowel 10-15 years earlier. The best available evidence suggests that only 10% of 1cm adenomas become malignant after 10 years. The incidence of adenomatous polyps in the colon increases with age, and although adenomatous polyps can be identified in about 20% of the population, most of these are small and unlikely to undergo malignant change. The vast majority (90%) of adenomas can be removed at colonoscopy, obviating the need for surgery. Other types of polyps occurring in the colon— such as metaplastic (or hyperplastic) polyps—are usually small and are much less likely than adenomas to become malignant.

Colorectal cancer is therefore a common condition, with a known premalignant lesion (adenoma). As it takes a relatively long time for malignant transformation from adenoma to carcinoma, and outcomes are markedly improved by early detection of adenomas and early cancers, the potential exists to reduce disease mortality through screening asymptomatic individuals for adenomas and early cancers.

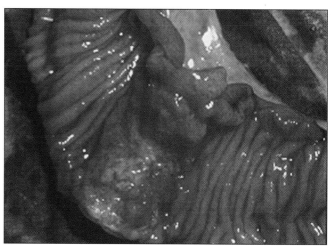

Figure 4.1 Colon cancer

Which screening test for population screening?

Education about bowel cancer is poor. A survey in 1991 showed that only 30% of the British population were aware that cancer of the bowel could occur. Such ignorance only adds to the difficulties of early detection for this form of cancer.

For a screening test to be applicable to large populations it has to be inexpensive, reliable, and acceptable. Many different screening tests for detecting early colorectal cancer have been tried. The simplest and least expensive is a questionnaire about symptoms, but this has proved predictably insensitive and becomes reliable only when the tumour is relatively advanced. Digital rectal examination and rigid sigmoidoscopy both suffer from the limitation that they detect only rectal or rectosigmoid cancers and are unpleasant and invasive.

Flexible sigmoidoscopy

Flexible sigmoidoscopy can detect 80% of colorectal cancers as it examines the whole of the left colon and rectum. A strategy of providing single flexible sigmoidoscopy for adults aged 55-65 years—with the aim of detecting adenomas—may be cost effective. A multicentre trial of this strategy for population screening is currently under evaluation.

Although flexible sigmoidoscopy is more expensive than rigid sigmoidoscopy, it is generally more acceptable to patients (it is less uncomfortable) and has much higher yield than the

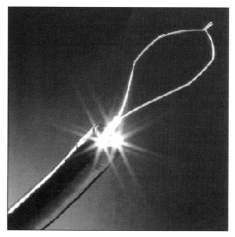

Figure 4.2 Flexible sigmoidoscope: used for endoluminal visualisation and therapeutic removal of adenomas

rigid instrument. Many nurses are now trained to perform flexible sigmoidoscopy, making potential screening programmes using this technique more cost effective. In a population screening programme, uptake of the offer of the screening test is crucial. Uptake is likely to be around 45%, and, of these, 6% will subsequently need full colonoscopy. The effect that this will have on the incidence of and mortality from colorectal cancer is uncertain until the completion of the multicentre trial in 2003.

Colonoscopy

Colonoscopy is the gold standard technique for examination of the colon and rectum, but its expense, the need for full bowel preparation and sedation, and the small risk of perforation of the colon make it unacceptable for population screening. Colonoscopy is, however, the investigation of choice for screening high risk patients (those at risk of hereditary non-polyposis colon cancer or with longstanding ulcerative colitis).

Barium enema

Barium enema, like colonoscopy, examines the whole colon and rectum, and, although it is cheaper and has a lower complication rate than colonoscopy, it is invasive and requires full bowel preparation. Whereas colonoscopy may be therapeutic (polypectomy), barium enema does not allow removal or biopsy of lesions seen. There are no population screening studies using barium enema.

Faecal occult blood tests

Faecal occult blood tests are the most extensively studied screening tests for colorectal cancer. These tests detect haematin from partially digested blood in the stool. Their overall sensitivity for colorectal neoplasia is only 50-60%, though their specificity is high. In screening studies of faecal occult blood tests, individuals are invited to take two samples from each of three consecutive stools. Compliance is around 50-60%, but with population education this might be improved. Individuals with more than four out of six positive tests (about 2% of participants) need colonoscopy.

Several large randomised studies have shown that screening with faecal occult blood testing is feasible, and two studies have shown that such screening reduces the mortality from colorectal cancer. In a study in Nottingham, for every 100 individuals with a positive test result, 12 had cancer and 23 had adenomatous polyps. The cancers detected at screening tended to be at an earlier stage than those presenting symptomatically (Dukes's A classification: 26% screen detected v 11% in controls). The disadvantage of screening with faecal occult bloods is its relatively low sensitivity—a third to a half of cancers will be missed on each round of screening. The Nottingham data suggest that screening every two years detects only 72% of cancers. This could be improved by testing annually and using more sensitive immunologically based faecal occult blood tests.

Who should be screened?

Although about 20% of the population will develop adenomatous polyps, only 5% of these will develop colorectal cancer. This equates to a 1 in 20 lifetime risk for colorectal cancer. The cancer occurs most often in the age group 65-75 years, but for adenomas the peak incidence is in a slightly earlier age group (55-65 years). Thus population screening for colorectal cancer should target both these age groups.

In addition, some people inherit a much higher susceptibility to colorectal cancer. Some inherit a well

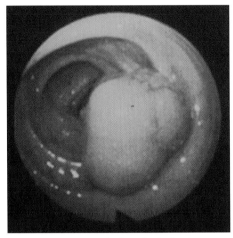

Figure 4.3 Colonoscopic view of colonic adenoma (about 1.5 cm diameter)

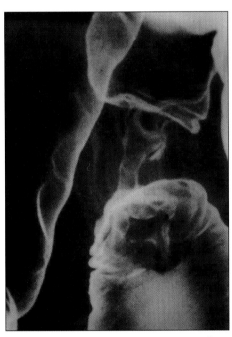

Figure 4.4 Double contrast barium enema showing carcinoma of sigmoid colon

---

Box 4.1 CT colography

- CT (computed tomographic) colography—virtual colonoscopy—is a new radiological technique that may have a role in population screening
- Although it requires full bowel preparation, highly expensive computed tomography scanners, and computing facilities, it is minimally invasive, and views of the whole colon can be obtained in five minutes
- Preliminary data suggest that this technique is as sensitive as colonoscopy or barium enema for detecting large polyps and cancers
- As yet, no trials of CT colography in population screening have been published
- CT colography has the potential to be cost effective and to reduce the need for colonoscopy in population screening

---

recognised single gene disorder, such as familial adenomatous polyposis or hereditary non-polyposis colon cancer, whereas most inherit an undetermined genetic abnormality. These people tend to develop colorectal cancer before the age of 50, and therefore screening in this high risk population needs to be tailored to each individual's risk pattern. They may also be at risk for cancers at other sites, and screening for ovarian, breast, and endometrial cancers may be appropriate in some of these cases. The advice of clinical geneticists in these cases can be invaluable.

Cost effectiveness of screening

If screening for colorectal cancer is to be acceptable to healthcare providers it must be shown to be cost effective. Estimates of the cost of screening for colorectal cancer range from £1000 to £3000 per life year saved, depending on the screening technique used. The cost of using faecal occult blood testing would be the lowest—similar to estimates for breast cancer screening.

Cost estimates are associated with several unknown factors. The factors that cause greatest concern to those considering funding screening programmes are the cost of cancers missed and the potential damage caused to asymptomatic individuals by invasive procedures such as colonoscopy.

Potential harm from screening

Although it has been suggested that considerable anxiety and psychological morbidity may be caused by inviting populations to participate in screening for colorectal cancer, little evidence exists to substantiate this. Indeed in the Nottingham trial no longstanding psychological morbidity from the screening programme was found. Similarly, no evidence exists that screening for colorectal cancer leads to false reassurance from negative tests.

Complications from colonoscopy (perforation and haemorrhage), however, can occur. The incidence of these complications is around 1 in 2000 procedures, and complications usually occur in therapeutic colonoscopy (endoscopic polypectomy) rather than in diagnostic procedures. Mortality from such events is rare.

Conclusions

- Screening for colorectal cancer using faecal occult blood tests is feasible; increasingly compelling evidence shows that such programmes can save lives at a cost similar to that of the existing breast cancer screening programme
- Once-only flexible sigmoidoscopy presents a promising alternative to faecal occult blood screening, but conclusive data will not be available for about five years
- For a screening programme to operate in the United Kingdom, considerable investment in colonoscopy facilities and expertise would be needed
- Several countries, including the United States, have screening programmes that use faecal occult blood tests or once-only flexible sigmoidoscopy, or both of these procedures. The United Kingdom has undertaken a pilot study in three areas to determine the feasibility of delivering a practicable, population based screening programme

Box 4.2 Inherited risk of colorectal cancer

High risk
- Familial adenomatous polyposis
- Hereditary non-polyposis colon cancer

Medium risk
- One first degree relative with colorectal cancer presenting at <45 years
- Two or more first degree relatives with colorectal cancer

Low risk
- Only one first degree relative with colorectal cancer presenting at >55 years
- No family history of colorectal cancer

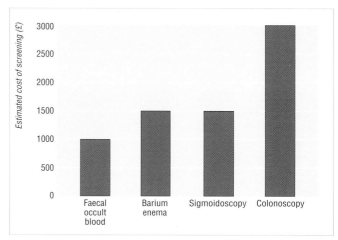

Figure 4.5 Estimates of costs for different methods of screening for colorectal cancer. Costs are based on biennial testing (faecal occult blood), testing at intervals of 5 years (barium enema and colonoscopy), or once-only testing (sigmoidoscopy)

Further reading

- Young GP, Rozen P, Levin B, eds. *Prevention and early detection of colorectal cancer.* London: Saunders, 1996.
- Kune G, ed. *Causes and control of colorectal cancer—a model for cancer prevention.* Boston, MA: Kluer Academic Publishers, 1996.
- Hardcastle JD, Chamberlain JO, Robinson MHE, Moss SM, Amar SA, Balfour TW, et al. Randomised controlled trial of faecal-occult-blood screening in colorectal cancer. *Lancet* 1996;348:1472-7.
- Mandel JS, Bond JH, Church TR, Snover DC, Bradley GM, Schuman LM, et al. Reducing mortality from colorectal cancer by screening for faecal occult blood. *N Engl J Med* 1993;328:1365-71.
- Winawer SJ, Schottenfield D, Felhinger BJ. Colorectal cancer screening. *J Natl Cancer Inst* 1991;83:243-53.

The picture of the flexible sigmoidoscope is published with permission from Endoscopy Support Services.

5 The role of primary care

F D Richard Hobbs

Every general practitioner in the United Kingdom will on average see one new case of colorectal cancer each year. For most primary care doctors the most important contributions they make to the care of patients with colorectal cancer relate to early diagnosis of the condition (including the point of referral) and to palliation of symptoms in those with established disease. Further roles in the future primary care service are screening for colorectal cancer (possibly using faecal occult blood testing) and a greater involvement in monitoring patients after curative procedures.

Early diagnosis and referral guidelines

Early diagnosis of colorectal cancer is essential in view of the stage related prognosis. Three potential levels of delay occur in the diagnosis of the disease: delay by the patient in presenting to the general practitioner; delay in referral by the general practitioner to a specialist; and delay by the hospital in either establishing the diagnosis or starting treatment. Detrimental differences between England and Wales and the rest of western Europe in survival rates for colorectal cancer arise primarily in the first six months after diagnosis, suggesting that these differences relate to late presentations or delays in treatment.

Patients presenting with symptoms

Most patients developing colorectal cancer will eventually present with symptoms. Primary symptoms include rectal bleeding persistently without anal symptoms and change in bowel habit—most commonly, increased frequency or looser stools (or both)—persistently over six weeks. Secondary effects include severe iron deficiency anaemia and clear signs of intestinal obstruction. Clinical examination may show a definite right sided abdominal mass or definite rectal mass.

Unfortunately, many large bowel symptoms are common and non-specific and often present late. Recently published guidelines, however, make specific recommendations about which patients should be urgently referred—within two weeks—for further investigation in the NHS. The guidelines also indicate which symptoms are highly unlikely to be caused by colorectal cancer.

The risk of colorectal cancer in young people is low (99% occurs in people aged over 40 years and 85% in those aged over 60). In patients aged under 45, therefore, initial management will depend on whether they have a family history of colorectal cancer—namely, a first degree relative (brother, sister, parent, or child) with colorectal cancer presenting below the age of 55, or two or more affected second degree relatives. Patients aged under 45 presenting with alarm symptoms and a family history of the disease should also be urgently referred for further investigation.

In patients suspected of having colorectal cancer, referral should be indicated as urgent (with an appointment expected within two weeks); the referral letter should include any relevant family history and details about symptoms and risk factors. An increasing number of general practitioners will have direct access to investigations, often via a rapid access rectal bleeding clinic. The usual investigations needed will be flexible colonoscopy or barium enema studies.

As colorectal cancer is the sixth most common cause of mortality in the United Kingdom, a general practitioner will on average care for a patient dying from colorectal cancer every 18 months

---

Box 5.1 Guidelines for urgent referral of patients with suspected colorectal cancer based on symptoms presented*

These combinations of symptoms and signs, when occurring for the first time, should be used to identify patients for urgent referral (that is, within two weeks). Patients need not have all symptoms

All ages
- Definite, palpable, right sided, abdominal mass
- Definite, palpable, rectal (not pelvic) mass
- Rectal bleeding with change in bowel habit to more frequent defecation or looser stools (or both) persistent over six weeks
- Iron deficiency anaemia (haemoglobin concentration < 110 g/l in men or < 100 g/l in postmenopausal women) without obvious cause

Age over 60 years (maximum age threshold could be 55 or 50)
- Rectal bleeding persistently without anal symptoms (soreness, discomfort, itching, lumps, prolapse, pain)
- Change of bowel habit to more frequent defecation or looser stools (or both), without rectal bleeding, and persistent for six weeks

*Adapted from the NHS Executive's *Referral Guidelines for Suspected Cancer* (London: Department of Health, 2000)

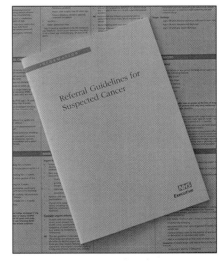

Figure 5.1 The NHS Executive's *Referral Guidelines for Suspected Cancer*

Box 5.2 Symptoms associated with low risk of malignancy*

Patients with the following symptoms but with no abdominal or rectal mass are at very low risk of colorectal cancer
- Rectal bleeding with anal symptoms (soreness, discomfort, itching, lumps, prolapse, pain)
- Change in bowel habit to less frequent defecation and harder stools
- Abdominal pain without clear evidence of intestinal obstruction

*Adapted from *Referral Guidelines for Suspected Cancer*

In the absence of a family history of the disease, younger patients with a negative physical examination, including a digital rectal examination, can be initially treated symptomatically. If symptoms persist, however, patients should be considered for further investigation.

Patients with genetic predisposition

All patients registering with a practice for the first time should provide details of their medical history. Patients with a history of familial adenomatous polyposis should be referred for DNA testing after the age of 15. Familial adenomatous polyposis accounts for about 1% of cases of colorectal cancer, with the defect gene identified on chromosome 5. Patients with a positive result should enter a programme of surveillance with flexible sigmoidoscopy.

The second common genetic predisposition to colorectal cancer is hereditary non-polyposis colon cancer. This condition should be suspected in patients describing three or more cases of colorectal cancer (or andenocarcinoma of the uterus) within their family. Such patients should be referred for endoscopic screening at the age of 25. Genetic testing for this condition is currently not feasible.

In patients with a first degree relative with colorectal cancer aged under 45 or with two first degree relatives with the disease, the lifetime risk of the cancer rises to over 1 in 10. Such patients should be referred for lower endoscopy screening once they are 10 years younger than the age at which the disease was diagnosed in the youngest affected relative. An earlier article in this series gives more detail on the genetics of colorectal cancer.

Population screening in primary care

The United Kingdom currently has no national screening programme for colorectal cancer. Several studies in the United States and Europe have shown that screening with faecal occult blood testing will reduce the overall mortality of colorectal cancer by about 15%. Such testing is a fairly simple procedure: only two small samples from different sites of a stool need to be collected on each of three consecutive days. In the United States, the specimens are then normally hydrated, whereas research in the United Kingdom and Denmark advocates using dry samples. The latter technique results in a lower sensitivity, but higher specificity—desirable test performance characteristics for an asymptomatic population screening procedure.

Faecal occult blood testing is therefore a cheap and easy method of screening, with reasonable levels of acceptability to the population. The main disadvantages of this test are the low sensitivity—with about 40% of cancers missed by a single screen, leading to the need for frequent faecal occult blood tests—and the fact that bleeding tends to occur late in the development of the disease. Furthermore there are no direct studies to guide on the most cost effective method of establishing a national screening programme using faecal occult blood testing. However, evidence from the cervical screening programme suggests that general practice led "call/recall" programmes would have the greatest impact.

A large Medical Research Council trial is currently evaluating once-only flexible sigmoidoscopy as a method of screening patients aged 50-60 years. The results of this trial will not be available for several years.

The American Cancer Society recommends an annual digital rectal examination for people aged over 40, an annual faecal occult blood test for people aged over 50, and flexible sigmoidoscopy every three to five years for people aged over 50. More detail on screening for colorectal cancer appears in an earlier article in this series.

Most (85-90%) colorectal cancers arise in people with no known risk factors, so opportunistic asymptomatic screening is of little value in colorectal cancer

---

Box 5.3 Patients with iron deficiency

- Patients aged 45 and over presenting with iron deficiency anaemia should be investigated to determine the cause of anaemia
- This will normally require both upper and lower bowel endoscopy
- In patients aged under 45, the cause of the anaemia should also be established, although the likelihood of this being colorectal cancer is low

---

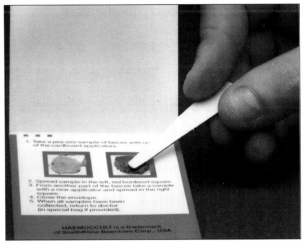

Figure 5.2 Haemoccult (SmithKline Beecham) has been the faecal occult blood test most often used in studies of the feasibility of screening for colorectal cancer

---

Table 5.1 Results from European population colorectal cancer screening trials using faecal occult blood testing kits (Haemoccult)

	Funen, Denmark (1985-95)	Nottingham, UK (1985-91)
Uptake (% of population screened)	67 (>92 in later rounds)	57 (range in general practices 29-74)
% of positive tests (range in rounds)	1-1.8 (n=215-261)	1.9-2.1 (n=837-924)
No of cases of colorectal cancer*	37/215, 25/261	83/837, 22/924
No of cases of adenomas (>10 mm)*	68/215, 56/261	311/837, 304/924
% predictive value for neoplasia	38-58	44-47
% predictive value for cancer	25-37	10-12 (17 for late responders)
% of patients with Dukes's A classification†:		
Intervention group	22	20
Control group	11	11
% of patients with Dukes's C and D classification†:		
Intervention group	39	46
Control group	47	52

*Funen: rounds 1 and 5; Nottingham: first screen and rescreen.
†P<0.01 for intervention versus control, both in Funen trial and in Nottingham trial.

Managing patients with established disease

After confirmation of diagnosis, the role of the primary care doctor revolves around advice, support, possibly monitoring for recurrence, and palliative care. Some general practices are involved with home based chemotherapy, usually coordinated by specialist outreach nurses.

In the United Kingdom primary care does not currently have a formal role in monitoring for disease recurrence after curative treatments. Data on this option are limited (see a later article in this series) but suggest that such surveillance could be safely conducted in primary care. Ideally, this monitoring should be accompanied by adequate infrastructure and training in primary care, with good liaison between the practice and secondary (or tertiary) care.

Limited evidence from other types of shared care indicate that certain factors are likely to improve outcomes: structured and planned discharge policies; the use of shared (preferably patient held) cards that document patient information (disease progress and drug treatments, as a minimum); locally agreed guidelines specifying the appropriate follow up and delineating responsibilities; and access to rapid referral clinics. As with follow up in all chronic diseases, the more communication between doctors and with the patients (and their families), the better the quality of care.

Where appropriate, the doctor should also counsel patients on any possible familial risk and the need for genetic counselling of relatives. The primary care doctor may also advise patients with diagnosed colorectal cancer about practical considerations, including access to social security benefits. In the United Kingdom eligibility for attendance allowance may be immediately available in the exceptional circumstance of cancer with a short terminal prognosis of less than six months.

For some patients, especially those with rectal tumours, the diagnosis of cancer is also accompanied by the necessity for either colostomy or ileostomy. Such patients will often require further specialised support, and liaison between the primary care team and specialist stoma nurses is important.

As the disease progresses, management will shift towards palliative care. Ideally, this would be delivered jointly by the primary care team and specialist palliative care services, such as those based at a hospice or provided by Macmillan nurses. Few data exist to guide on the most effective models for palliative care in colorectal cancer. However, non-randomised studies have shown high satisfaction among patients when they are kept fully involved in understanding the progression of their disease and their treatment options, when shared care cards are used, and when home care teams are provided.

The main priorities in palliative care in colorectal cancer include the management of pain, jaundice, ascites, constipation, and nausea. The importance of attempting to correct these symptoms cannot be overstated: as much distress may be caused by constipation or nausea as by pain. Full explanations of signs such as jaundice are likely to be reassuring. Moreover, the advent of specialist home care teams (with access to specialist equipment—such as bed aids to preserve pressure areas or syringe drivers for pain control) and skilled counsellors for patients and their families, enables virtually all patients who wish it to remain at home.

Such an option is further enhanced by relief admission—when necessary for the patient or the family—to specialist palliative care wards or, more likely, to a hospice. In the United Kingdom only a minority of patients with colorectal cancer currently die from their disease in hospital or in a hospice.

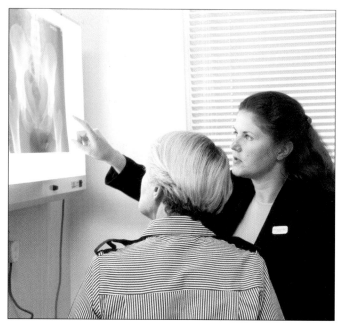

Figure 5.3 Macmillan nurses have an important role in community palliative care, liaising with both professionals and patients

Further reading

- Carter S, Winslet M. Delay in the presentation of colorectal cancer: a review of causation. *Int J Colorectal Dis* 1998;13(1):27-31.
- Crossland A, Jones R. Rectal bleeding: prevalence and consultation behaviour. *BMJ* 1995;311:486-8.
- Curless R, French J, Williams G, James O. Comparison of gastro-intestinal symptoms in colorectal carcinoma patients and community control to the respect of age. *Gut* 1994;35:1267-70.
- Fijten GH, Starmans R, Muris JW, Schouten HJ, Blijham GH, Knottnerus J. Predictive value of signs and symptoms for colorectal cancer in patients with rectal bleeding in general practice. *Fam Pract* 1995;12:279-86.
- Hardcastle JD, Chamberlain JO, Robinson MHE, Moss SM, Amar SS, Balfour TW, et al. Randomised controlled trial of faecal-occult-blood screening for colorectal cancer. *Lancet* 1996;348:1472-7.
- Hobbs FDR, Cherry RC, Fielding JWL, Pike L, Holder R. Acceptability of opportunistic screening for occult gastrointestinal blood loss. *BMJ* 1992;304:483-6.
- Kronborg O, Olsen J, Jorgensen O, Sondergaard O. Randomised study of screening for colorectal cancer with faecal-occult blood test. *Lancet* 1996;348:1467-71.
- Spurgeon P, Barwell F, Kerr D. Waiting times for cancer patients in England after general practitioners' referrals: retrospective national survey. *BMJ* 2000;320:838-9.
- St John DJ, McDermott FT, Hopper JL, Debney EA, Johnson WR, Hughes ES. Cancer risk in relatives of patients with common colorectal cancer. *Ann Intern Med* 1993;118:785-90.

The photograph of the Macmillan nurses is published with permission from Macmillan Cancer Relief.

6 Primary treatment—does the surgeon matter?

Colin McArdle

The dominant factor contributing to the relatively poor prognosis for colorectal cancer is the advanced stage of the disease at the time of initial presentation: up to a third of patients have locally advanced or metastatic disease, which precludes surgical cure. Even in the patients who undergo apparently curative resection, almost half die within five years.

In the west of Scotland, for example, about a third of 1842 patients presenting with colorectal cancer to seven hospitals between 1991 and 1994 presented as emergencies. Potentially curative resection was achieved in about 70% of patients presenting electively; the curative resection rate was lower in those presenting as emergencies. Five per cent of patients admitted for elective surgery and 13% of those admitted as emergencies died. Almost 60% of elective patients survived two years, compared with 44% of patients admitted as emergencies. These results are typical of population based studies in the United Kingdom.

Variation among surgeons

Most surgeons acknowledge that the incidence of postoperative complications varies widely among individual surgeons. It is now almost 20 years since Fielding and his colleagues in the large bowel cancer project drew attention to differences in anastomotic leak and local recurrence rates after resection for large bowel cancer.

In the original Glasgow Royal Infirmary study, which was conducted in the 1980s, similar differences in postoperative morbidity and mortality were noted. Furthermore, after apparently curative resection, survival at 10 years varied threefold among surgeons.

One might argue that these are historical data and therefore bear little relevance to the current situation. In the current west of Scotland study, however, although overall 33% of patients presented as emergencies, the proportion varied among hospitals from 24% to 41% and among surgeons from 10% to 50%.

Similarly, the proportion of patients undergoing curative resection varied among surgeons from 45% to 82%; postoperative mortality, in patients presenting electively, also varied, from 0% to 17%. Several out of the 16 surgeons studied performed less well than their colleagues.

Several factors apart from the individual surgeon's skill might influence these measurements of immediate and long

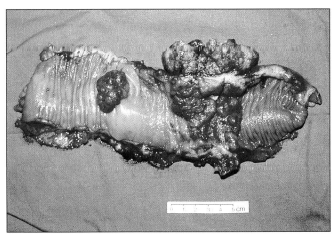

Figure 6.1 Colorectal adenoma and tumour—does a patient's survival depend on which surgeon operates?

Table 6.2 Variation in outcome, by surgeon, after curative resection (n=338)

	Overall rate (%)	Range among surgeons (%)
Anastomotic leak	9	0-25
Local recurrence	11	0-21
Postoperative mortality	6	0-20
Survival (10 years)	41	20-63

Data are from the original Glasgow Royal Infirmary study (McArdle et al, *BMJ* 1991;302:1501-5)

Table 6.1 Presentation, type of surgery, and postoperative mortality, by hospital and surgeon (n=1842), west of Scotland study. Values are percentages

	All (mean)	Hospital (range)	Surgeon (range)
Emergency admission	33	24-41	10-50
Dukes's classification A or B	49	43-56	29-68
Curative resection	68	63-75	45-82
Palliative resection	25	15-29	11-48
Postoperative mortality:			
Elective	5	0-7	0-17
Emergency	13	9-24	4-38

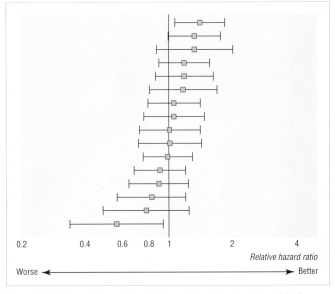

Figure 6.2 95% confidence intervals for relative risk of outcome, for all resections, by surgeon (n=16), west of Scotland study

term outcome: case mix; surgical philosophy; assessment of cure; quality of pathological reporting; other prognostic factors; small numbers (see box). Despite these factors it seems likely that the differences in the immediate postoperative morbidity and mortality observed among surgeons in the above studies are genuine. There have now been several analyses of immediate outcome after colorectal cancer surgery, and in each study, the results have been broadly comparable.

Effect of volume of surgery

Two explanations are possible for the differences in outcome among surgeons—namely, the number of patients treated by individual surgeons and whether these surgeons are specialists.

Although good evidence exists for other types of surgery that volume of work is important, in colorectal cancer convincing evidence that volume affects outcome is lacking. In the Lothian and Borders study, 5 of 20 consultants were responsible for 50% of the rectal cancer procedures. These five surgeons had a significantly lower anastomotic leak rate, but this may reflect specialisation rather than volume of work. In the German multicentre study, a group of surgeons with low work volume and performing only a few rectal cancer procedures had local recurrence rates well within the range of results obtained by individual surgeons with high work loads. Furthermore, in a recent analysis of outcome in 927 patients treated in the Manchester area, after correction for non-prognostic variables no relation between volume and outcome was noted.

Role of specialisation

The question of specialisation is more complex. Clearly rectal cancer surgery represents a greater technical challenge than colonic surgery. It therefore seems reasonable to expect—but it is remarkably difficult to show (largely because of the small numbers of patients treated by individual surgeons)—that specialist surgeons achieve better outcome. Analysis of outcome in almost 1400 patients with rectal cancer randomised in the Swedish preoperative radiotherapy studies, suggested that local recurrence and death rates were significantly lower in those patients operated on by surgeons with more than 10 years' experience as a specialist.

Perhaps the best information, however, comes from the Canadian study in which 683 patients with rectal cancer were treated by 52 different surgeons, five of whom were trained in colorectal surgery. These five surgeons performed 109 (16%) of the procedures. Independent of the type of training received by the surgeons, 323 procedures (47%) were performed by surgeons who each did fewer than 21 resections over the study period. Multivariate analysis showed that the risk of local recurrence was increased in patients treated both by surgeons not trained in colorectal surgery and by surgeons performing fewer than 21 resections. Similarly, disease specific survival was lower in the patients treated by these two groups of surgeons. These results suggest that both specialisation and volume may be important independent factors determining outcome.

Surgeons are currently under intense scrutiny, partly because readily available measures of outcome exist and partly because outcome seems to differ substantially among surgeons. The issues, however, are complex. Small numbers, annual accounting, and failure to take into account case mix, surgical intent, quality of staging, and prognostic factors may lead to inappropriate conclusions.

Box 6.1 Influences, apart from surgeon's skill, on immediate and long term outcome of colorectal surgery

Case mix
Non-specialist surgeons tend to have a high proportion of elderly patients, often with concomitant disease, who present as emergencies with advanced lesions; specialist surgeons may have fewer emergencies, with most patients being younger, fitter, and with less advanced disease

Surgical philosophy
Faced with the same problem, an aggressive surgeon might undertake radical surgery, thereby risking technical complications, in an attempt to improve quality and duration of life, whereas a conservative surgeon might opt for limited surgery, thereby minimising the risk of postoperative complications (but in doing so, he or she may compromise long term survival)

Assessment of cure
The decision on whether a resection is curative or palliative is often based on the surgeon's subjective impression at the time of laparotomy. In patients in whom the adequacy of resection was borderline an optimistic surgeon might believe a cure had been achieved, whereas a more pessimistic surgeon might believe that only palliation had been achieved

Quality of pathological reporting
Limited sampling might suggest that the lymph nodes and the lateral resection margins were clear of tumour, whereas more rigorous sampling might show the presence of more extensive disease. The resultant pathological stage migration might therefore alter expectation of outcome and lead to in inappropriate interpretation of the results

Other prognostic factors
Other factors—for example, socioeconomic deprivation—should be taken into consideration

Small numbers
Most surgeons at times have a cluster of patients who do less well than expected. This will vary from year to year. Any conclusion based on a small sample is likely to be misleading as it pertains to the individual surgeon

---

Table 6.3 Local recurrence and disease specific survival (n=683), according to specialisation and volume of work. Values are percentages

Training in colorectal surgery	Surgeons performing <21 resections (323 procedures)	Surgeons performing ≥21 resections (360 procedures)
No (n = 574):		
Local recurrence	44.6	27.8
Survival	39.2	49
Yes (n = 109):		
Local recurrence	21.1	10.4
Survival	54.5	67.3

Data are from the Canadian study (Porter et al, *Ann Surg* 1998;227:157-67)

Even if confounding variables are taken into account, some surgeons seem to be less competent than others, with poorer outcomes

Nevertheless, the results of the studies discussed here suggest that some surgeons are less competent than their colleagues and that these factors may compromise survival. Considerable effort and resources are currently being poured into large multicentre studies of adjuvant chemotherapy and radiotherapy in an effort to provide a marginal improvement in the survival of patients with colorectal cancer. If, by specialisation, the overall results of surgery could be improved—and evidence suggests that this is so—the impact on survival might be greater than that of any of the adjuvant therapies currently under study.

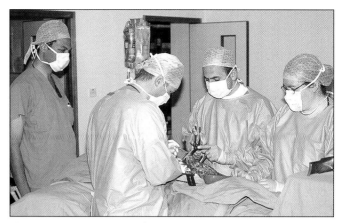

Figure 6.3 Outcome seems to differ substantially among surgeons performing colorectal surgery—specialisation rather than volume of work might be a way of improving overall outcome

Further reading
- Holm T, Johansson H, Cedermark B, Ekelund G, Rutqvist L-E. Influence of hospital and surgeon related factors and outcome after treatment of rectal cancer with or without pre-operative radiotherapy. *Br J Surg* 1997;87:657-63.
- McArdle CS, Hole D. Impact of variability among surgeons on post-operative morbidity and mortality and ultimate survival. *BMJ* 1991;302:1501-5.
- Parry JM, Collins S, Mathers J, Scott NA, Woodman CBJ. Influence of volume of work on the outcome of treatment for patients with colorectal cancer. *Br J Surg* 1998;86:475-81.
- Porter GA, Soskolne CL, Yakimets WW, Newman SC. Surgeon-related factors and outcome in rectal cancer. *Ann Surg* 1998;227:157-67.

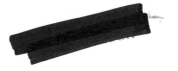

7 Adjuvant therapy

Rachel S J Midgley, D J Kerr

Despite substantial improvements in surgical technique and postoperative care, colorectal cancer continues to kill 95 000 people in Europe alone each year.

Of the annual 150 000 newly diagnosed cases, about 80% have no macroscopic evidence of residual tumour after resection. More than half of patients, however, develop recurrence and die of their disease. This is a result of occult viable tumour cells that have metastasised before surgery and which are undetectable by current radiological techniques (the limit of detection of standard computed tomography is about $1cm^3$, equivalent to 10^9 cells).

Adjuvant treatment (chemotherapy and radiotherapy) has developed as an auxiliary weapon to surgery and is aimed at eradicating these micrometastatic cancer cells before they become established and refractory to intervention. As the presence of the primary tumour can exert an inhibitory influence on micrometastases, theoretically the removal of the tumour might stimulate growth of any residual cells, increasing the proliferating fraction and rendering them more susceptible to the cytotoxic effects of the widely used cytotoxic agent, fluorouracil.

It is reasonable to predict therefore that the earlier chemotherapy is started after surgery, the greater the potential benefit, although this has not yet been formally addressed in adjuvant trials. Implicit in this belief is a necessity for a multidisciplinary effort between surgeon, oncologist, and the community care team to provide seamless, streamlined cancer care for the individual patient.

Pharmacology of fluorouracil

Fluorouracil has remained the cornerstone chemotherapy for colorectal cancer for over 40 years. It is a prodrug that is converted intracellularly to various metabolites that bind to the enzyme thymidylate synthase, inhibiting synthesis of thymidine, DNA, and RNA. Increasing understanding of the molecular pharmacology of fluorouracil has led to the development of strategies to increase its efficacy.

The first strategy to be tested was coadministration with the immunostimulatory, antihelminthic drug levamisole, but despite promising early results, recent trials have not convincingly shown significant improvements in outcome compared with fluorouracil alone. In addition, no persuasive mechanism for the assumed synergism between fluorouracil and levamisole has been found.

In contrast, addition of folinic acid increases and prolongs the inhibition of the target enzyme (thymidylate synthase) and seems to confer improved clinical outcome compared with fluorouracil alone in advanced disease and when used in adjuvant therapy.

The side effects of chemotherapy based on fluorouracil vary according to the regimen (most commonly given as bolus intravenously daily for 5 days every 4 weeks or bolus weekly). They include nausea, vomiting, an increased susceptibility to infection, oral mucositis, diarrhoea, desquamation of the palms and soles, and, rarely, cardiac and neurological toxic effects.

Adjuvant—helpful, assisting, auxiliary (from Latin *ad* to, and *juvare* to help)

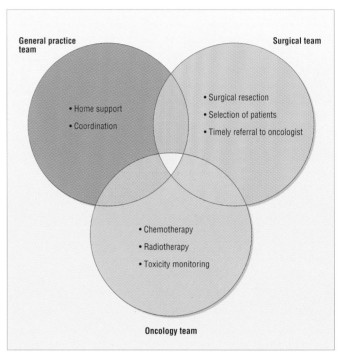

Figure 7.1 Optimising adjuvant therapy requires careful coordination between general practice, surgical, and oncology teams

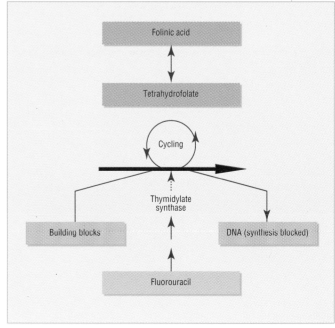

Figure 7.2 Intracellular metabolism and mechanism of action of fluorouracil and modulation by folinic acid

Established benefits of fluorouracil based adjuvant chemotherapy

Early adjuvant trials were retrospective and underpowered and failed to show any therapeutic benefit with respect to recurrence rate or survival. In 1990, however, the results of the intergroup trial were published. In this study 318 patients with stage B colorectal malignancy were randomised for surgical treatment alone or surgery followed by fluorouracil plus levamisole. In addition, 929 patients with stage C malignancy received surgery alone, surgery plus levamisole, or surgery plus fluorouracil and levamisole. For these patients there was a 33% reduction in the odds of death and a 41% decrease in recurrence among those treated with fluorouracil plus levamisole compared with surgery alone or surgery plus levamisole.

In contrast with levamisole, combining folinic acid with fluorouracil is pharmacologically rational, and documented benefit in advanced disease led to the logical extension of this combination into adjuvant therapy. Three large randomised adjuvant phase III trials produced confirmatory evidence of improved, disease-free survival at three years and improved overall survival in patients treated with fluorouracil plus folinic acid, with a 25-30% decrease in the odds of dying from colon cancer (or an absolute improvement in survival of 5-6% compared with controls).

Recently a meta-analysis of updated individual data from all unconfounded randomised studies of adjuvant chemotherapy (including the above three trials) has been undertaken (Colorectal Cancer Collaborative Group, unpublished). Overall, there was a 6-7% absolute improvement in survival with chemotherapy compared with surgery alone (SD 2.3, P = 0.01). The analysis advised that on current evidence the combination of fluorouracil plus folinic acid should be accepted as "standard" adjuvant chemotherapy for patients with Dukes's type C colon cancer.

Controversies in adjuvant therapy

Despite convincing evidence that adjuvant chemotherapy improves disease-free survival and overall survival in Dukes's type C colon cancer (an estimated six deaths prevented for 100 patients treated), several controversies surrounding the application of this form of treatment still exist.

Length of treatment and optimal dose of fluorouracil plus folinic acid

Lengthy adjuvant treatment has adverse effects on patients' quality of life as well as financial implications. A recent North American study, however, has shown that six months' treatment is as effective as 12 months'.

Determining the optimal dose is important: high dose folinic acid is 10 times as expensive as low dose. This issue has been addressed in the "certain" arm of the United Kingdom Co-ordinating Committee on Cancer Research's QUASAR ("quick and simple and reliable") trial (patients with Dukes's type C colon cancer). The trial uses the principle of randomising according to certain or uncertain indication: if, for a particular subgroup of patients the worth in receiving some form of adjuvant chemotherapy is definitely established from published randomised controlled trials (for example, patients with Dukes's type C colon cancer) then these patients are randomised to the certain indication arm (with a choice of different drugs and regimens); if, however, no definitive evidence exists of worth in a particular subgroup (for example, in patients with Dukes's type B colon cancer or with rectal

Table 7.1 Results of three international randomised controlled trials of adjuvant chemotherapy (fluorouracil plus folinic acid v control) for patients with colon cancer. Values are percentage survival and P values

Trial	Disease-free survival	Overall survival
Overview of French, Italian, and Canadian trials (n = 1493)*	71 v 62 (< 0.0001)	83 v 78 (0.03)
Intergroup study (n = 309)†	74 v 58 (0.004)	74 v 63 (0.02)
NSABP C-03 trial (n = 1080)‡	73 v 64 (0.0004)	84 v 77 (0.003)

NSABP C-03 = national surgical adjuvant breast and bowel project—colon (protocol No 3).
*Fluorouracil plus high dose folinic acid v observation alone, 3 year follow up.
†Fluorouracil plus low dose folinic acid v observation alone, 5 year follow up.
‡Fluorouracil plus high dose folinic acid v methylCCNU, oncovin, or fluorouracil.

Box 7.1 Controversies still surrounding adjuvant therapy

- For how long should adjuvant therapy be continued, and what is the optimal dose of fluorouracil plus folinic acid?
- What is the role of adjuvant chemotherapy in lower risk groups?
- Is adjuvant therapy useful in rectal cancer?
- What is the role of new agents (eg irinotecan and oxaliplatin)?

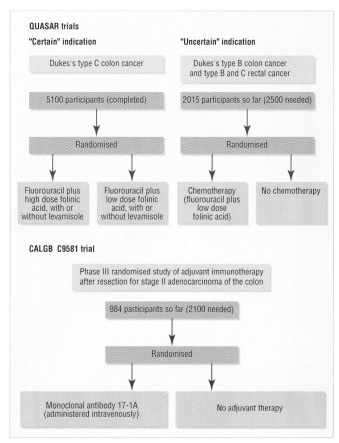

Figure 7.3 Ongoing adjuvant trials in colorectal cancer

cancer) then the patients are randomised into the uncertain indication arm (chemotherapy v no chemotherapy). The results from QUASAR's certain arm show that neither high dose folinic acid nor levamisole contribute to improved survvial.

Role of adjuvant chemotherapy in lower risk groups

Inadequate data exist on the effect of chemotherapy in stage B colon cancer. The proportional reduction in annual risk is probably similar for stage B and stage C patients. If the proportional reductions in mortality are similar, the absolute benefits in terms of five year survival would be somewhat smaller for stage B patients than for stage C patients because of lower risk of recurrence (perhaps two to three lives saved per 100 patients treated).

Patients with stage B cancers who have prognostic indicators that suggest a high risk of recurrence (for example, perforation, vascular invasion, poor differentiation) might benefit proportionately more than patients with stage B cancer without high risk indicators and these variables might define a subgroup of patients who might merit adjuvant chemotherapy. Little evidence exists, however, on the prognostic predictability of these various features.

Use of adjuvant therapy in rectal cancer

Insufficient evidence exists to support the routine use of systemic chemotherapy in either Dukes's type B or type C rectal cancer. Anatomical constraints make the rectum less accessible to the surgeon, so it is much more difficult to achieve wide excision of the tumour, and about 50% of recurrences are in the pelvis itself rather than at distant sites. This means that locally directed radiotherapy is a useful adjuvant weapon, and this has been assessed for rectal cancer both before and after surgery.

In the largest trial of preoperative radiotherapy (the Swedish rectal cancer trial), radiotherapy produced a 61% decrease in local recurrence and an improvement in overall survival (58% v 48%) compared with surgery alone. Radiotherapy after surgery seems to be less effective, even at higher doses, possibly because of rapid repopulation of tumour cells after surgery or relative hypoxia around the healing wound.

Only one trial, the Uppsala trial in Sweden, has directly compared radiotherapy before and after surgery. Despite a higher dose after surgery, a significant reduction occurred in local recurrence rates among patients treated before surgery (12% v 21%, P < 0.02).

Animal studies have suggested that fluorouracil may prime the tumour cells and increase the cytotoxic effect of subsequent radiotherapy. Some clinical data support the role of chemoradiotherapy combinations in rectal cancer, but further clinical evidence of benefit needs to be provided before this treatment could be considered for routine use. The uncertain arm of the QUASAR trial will help to resolve this issue.

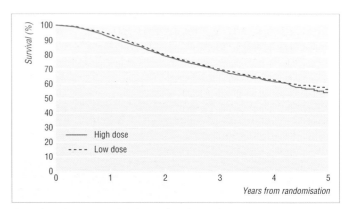

Figure 7.4 Five year survival for 4927 patients with colorectal cancer randomised to high dose or low dose folinic acid with fluorouracil

> **The uncertain arm of the QUASAR trial is aiming to establish whether chemotherapy is justified in Dukes's type B colon cancer and to define which factors might help to predict chemotherapeutic benefit**

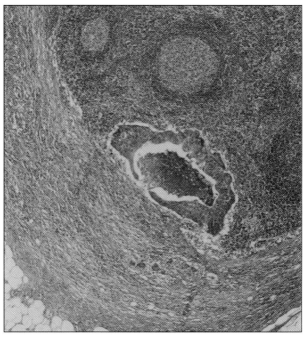

Figure 7.5 Microscopic metastasis in a draining lymph node from a rectal cancer

Table 7.2 Benefits of adjuvant therapy

Site and stage	Chemotherapy	Radiotherapy
Dukes's type C colon cancer	Worth established; fluorouracil plus folinic acid optimal to date; six lives per 100 treated saved; new drugs entering trial	No benefit
Dukes's type B colon cancer	Worth not established; particular subgroups of patients may benefit (on basis of histological and other prognostic factors)	No benefit
Dukes's type B or C rectal cancer	Worth not established	Worth established; preoperative may be superior to postoperative in terms of both efficacy and reducing toxicity

Role of portal venous infusional therapy

Fluorouracil is an S phase specific drug, and yet its active metabolites have a half life of about 10 minutes, which limits its target, when given as a bolus, to the small fraction of cells in the S phase at the time of administration. Infusional therapy can therefore affect a greater proportion of cells. In addition, the most common site for micrometastases after resection of a colorectal tumour is the liver. In contrast with macroscopically identifiable metastases of advanced disease, which derive their blood supply from the hepatic artery, these micrometastases are thought to be supplied by the portal vein. Therefore delivering chemotherapy via the portal vein should provide high concentrations of the drug at the most vulnerable site and lead to substantial first pass metabolism, which should attenuate any systemic toxicity. The established regimen for portal fluorouracil in adjuvant therapy is a course of 5-7 days starting immediately after surgery. A meta-analysis of 10 randomised trials showed a 4.7% improvement in absolute survival with portal venous infusion therapy compared with surgery alone; however, the confidence intervals were wide and the statistical benefit is not robust. Indeed the AXIS trial, the largest single trial of portal venous infusion to date, randomising 4000 patients after surgery either to the infusion therapy or to observation alone at five years, suggests no significant differences in overall survival.

Future role of adjuvant therapy

The use of adjuvant therapy in colorectal cancer over the past 40 years has centred on fluorouracil, alone and in combination, and on the fine tuning of regimen and route of administration. Current trials are considering new drugs (eg irinotecan and oxaliplatin) and their sequencing, as well as innovative techniques, such as immunotherapy and gene therapy. These techniques will be considered in detail later in the series. Gene therapy and immunotherapy are likely to function optimally, however, when cellular load is low, blood supply is good, and small clusters of cells are surrounded by effectors of the immune system; these therapies may therefore be most suitable as adjuvant therapy rather than for use in advanced disease.

All cytotoxic agents are rigorously tested and applied in advanced disease before being used in adjuvant therapy. New agents that are now entering adjuvant trials will be fully described in the next article in this series.

The United Kingdom Co-ordinating Committee on Cancer Research's AXIS study, in which 4000 patients have been randomised to portal vein infusion versus surgery alone, will contribute substantially to the debate on this type of therapy

---

Further reading

- Gray R. Adjuvant treatment for colorectal cancer. In: *Guidance on commissioning cancer services: improving outcomes in colorectal cancer.* London: Department of Health, 1997.
- Midgley RS, Kerr DJ. Adjuvant treatment of colorectal cancer. *Cancer Treat Rev* 1997;23:135-52.
- Midgley RS, Kerr DJ. Colorectal cancer. *Lancet* 1999;353:391-9.

The authors acknowledge the support of the Cancer Research Campaign and the Medical Research Council.

The survival graph is adpated from the *Lancet* (2000;355:1588-96); the illustration of microscopic metastasis was supplied by Dr D C Rowlands.

8 Treatment of advanced disease

Annie M Young, Daniel Rea

Advanced colorectal cancer can be defined as colorectal cancer that at presentation or recurrence is either metastatic or so locally advanced that surgical resection is unlikely to be carried out with curative intent. Despite most patients undergoing potentially curative surgery and the availability of adjuvant chemotherapy, about 50% of patients presenting with colorectal adenocarcinoma die from subsequent metastatic disease. The five year survival rate for advanced colorectal cancer is lower than 5%.

Clinical presentation

Local recurrence of a tumour is more common in rectal than colon primaries. It may be identified early in the asymptomatic phase by follow up monitoring or may present with similar symptoms to the primary lesion. Blood loss through the rectum, mucous discharge, altered bowel habit, and straining are common features of recurrent rectal cancer. Pain and urinary symptoms are features of localised pelvic recurrence. Recurrent intra-abdominal disease can present as small or large bowel obstruction, and recurrence at other sites may be indicated by focal features such as hepatic capsular pain, jaundice, dyspnoea, localised bone pain, or neurological symptoms. Systemic features of weight loss, anorexia, nausea, and asthenia are symptoms commonly associated with advanced colorectal cancer. The tumour is often palpable on rectal or abdominal examination, and malignant ascites may also be evident.

Referral

Despite clear evidence of the value of chemotherapy and the apparent willingness of cancer patients to have chemotherapy, in the United Kingdom only about 25% of patients with advanced disease are referred to an oncology tertiary centre for consideration of chemotherapy. Referral patterns and treatment policies for patients with advanced colorectal cancer vary widely in the United Kingdom. Currently many regions are in the throws of reorganising their cancer services as part of the implementation of the Calman report, *A Policy Framework for Commissioning Cancer Services*. It is envisaged that referrals to oncologists will increase considerably owing to the publication in 1997 of guidelines for managing colorectal cancer.

Overview of management

The management of patients with advanced colorectal cancer involves a combination of specialist active treatment, symptom control measures, and psychosocial support. Active treatment comprises an individual plan (often combining palliative surgery), cytotoxic chemotherapy, and radiation therapy.

The outcome measures of the impact of active treatment have traditionally been survival, response, and toxicity. Alternative end points—for example, quality of life, convenience, acceptability to patients, and patients' preferences—assume greater importance in those with advanced disease, and they should now also be incorporated into the assessment of the relative worth of treatments.

In the past few years several therapeutic advances—underpinned by multiprofessional, site specialised team working—have finally changed the view that advanced colorectal cancer is an untreatable disease. Although cytotoxic chemotherapy is not suitable for all patients, widespread use in appropriate situations can improve survival and quality of life

---

Box 8.1 Clinical presentation

- About 20% of colorectal cancer cases will present with advanced disease
- About 50% of patients treated with curative surgery will develop advanced disease
- About 80% of relapses will occur within three years of primary surgery
- About 50% of patients with advanced disease will present with liver metastasis
- About 20% of patients with advanced disease have disease confined to the liver

---

Box 8.2 Which patients should be referred for palliative chemotherapy*?

Patients in whom chemotherapy should be considered
- Able to carry out all normal activity without restriction
- Restricted in physically strenuous activity but able to walk about and carry out light work
- Able to walk about and capable of all self care but unable to carry out any work; out of bed or chair for more than 50% of waking hours

Patients unlikely to benefit from chemotherapy
- Capable only of limited self care; confined to bed or chair for more than 50% of waking hours
- Severely disabled; cannot carry out any self care; totally confined to bed or chair

*Based on the World Health Organization's criteria for functional performance status

---

Box 8.3 Current status of chemotherapy

- Many patients with advanced colorectal cancer die without having received chemotherapy
- Chemotherapy improves survival by an average of about six months, compared with supportive care alone
- Chemotherapy improves overall quality of life
- Stabilisation of disease with chemotherapy improves both survival and disease related symptoms
- Early chemotherapy treatment (rather than waiting until symptoms appear) prolongs survival

Surgery

Palliative surgical procedures for advanced colorectal cancer are commonly used to overcome obstructing lesions and to alleviate pelvic symptoms. The liver is the most frequent site of metastasis, and in selected patients with no extrahepatic metastases surgical resection offers the only hope of cure. Five year survival rates of 25-35% have been reported with this highly specialised procedure (Cady and Stone, 1991).

Radiotherapy

In advanced colon cancer, radiotherapy is rarely indicated. In locally advanced rectal disease, localised radiation may render some tumours resectable. Radiotherapy can also be effective in palliation of symptoms—it can improve pain, stop haemorrhage, and lessen straining. In the absence of distant metastases, radiation may afford long term control of the tumour. Pain from isolated bone metastases can also be alleviated with short courses of radiation.

Conventional chemotherapy

In patients with advanced colorectal cancer, chemotherapy is delivered with palliative rather than curative intent. For over four decades fluorouracil has been the mainstay of treatment for advanced colorectal cancer. Folinic acid is given intravenously before fluorouracil to enhance the fluorouracil's cytotoxicity. Large randomised trials of chemotherapy versus best supportive care have shown that fluorouracil based chemotherapy adds about 4-6 months to the remaining life of patients with advanced colorectal cancer. Chemotherapy delays the occurrence or progression of symptoms by about six months and improves symptoms, weight gain, and functional performance in about 40% of patients. Palliative chemotherapy in advanced colorectal cancer should not be restricted by chronological age but by fitness and activity level.

Is failure to respond a failure of treatment?
Less than a third of patients receive an objective tumour response—complete or partial—with fluorouracil based therapy. In a further 20-30% of patients, the disease is stabilised during chemotherapy. The patients with stable disease ("no change" category) also derive a symptomatic and survival advantage from chemotherapy.

Which regimen?
Current evidence supports the use of infusional fluorouracil regimens over bolus schedules in terms of both toxicity and efficacy, but infusional chemotherapy is more complex to administer, requiring permanent vascular access technology or admission to hospital. In the United Kingdom a 48 hour regimen of fluorouracil plus folinic acid repeated every 14 days is commonly used. Ideally, chemotherapy for advanced colorectal cancer should be given within the umbrella of a clinical trial to help resolve outstanding questions of optimal type, duration, and scheduling of therapy.

Tailoring treatment
The optimum duration of chemotherapy is unknown and is currently being tested in clinical trials. The current approaches are either to treat for a fixed period (usually six months) or to treat until progression occurs. Irrespective of which of these approaches is adopted, the overriding need is to monitor rigorously the effect of treatment in terms of response, palliative

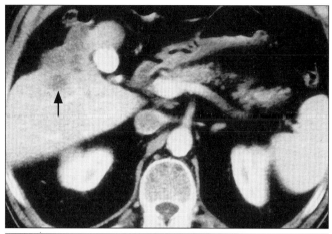

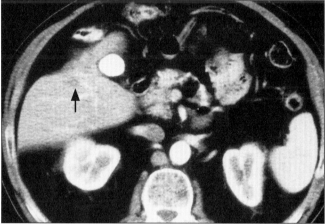

Figure 8.1 Abdominal computed tomogram showing a hepatic metastasis (arrow) before chemotherapy (top) and 17 weeks after chemotherapy (bottom); the later image shows a substantial reduction in the bulk of the hepatic tumour

---

Box 8.4 Definitions for assessing response and progression after chemotherapy

Complete response—Disappearance of all known disease, determined by two observations not less than four weeks apart

Partial response—Decrease of at least 50% of the sum of the products of the largest perpendicular diameters of all measurable lesions as determined by two observations not less than four weeks apart

No change—Less than 50% decrease and less than 25% increase in the sum of the products of the largest perpendicular diameters of all measurable lesions; no new lesions should appear

Progressive disease—More than 25% increase in the size of at least one lesion or appearance of a new lesion

---

Data from trials by the Nordic Gastrointestinal Tumour Therapy Group support the early use of chemotherapy, before the patient's condition deteriorates

benefit, and toxicity. This ensures that any toxicity or disease progression is recognised as soon as possible and that the appropriate individualised treatment or cessation of chemotherapy can be implemented without delay.

Chemotherapy toxicity

Chemotherapy for advanced colorectal cancer should be prescribed by experienced oncologists familiar with the toxicity profile of the drug regimens used. Despite concerns over toxicity, currently used infusional regimens are remarkably well tolerated. Management of toxicities in the community requires close liaison with the hospital team, and severe toxicity requires immediate admission. The most common effects of toxicity from chemotherapies for advanced colorectal cancer are diarrhoea, mucositis, asthenia, and neutropenia. Nausea, alopecia, and anorexia can also be experienced. Diarrhoea can be substantially relieved with oral antimotility drugs. Mucositis should be managed with antiseptic mouthwash and prophylactic or early treatment of oral candidiasis. Neutropenia is less common with current infusional regimens but must always be suspected in patients with fever. Prolonged treatment with fluorouracil can produce painful blistering erythema of palms and soles of the feet (palmar plantar erythrodysaesthesia), which often improves with pyridoxine.

Cost effectiveness

In 1995 Glimelius et al showed that the overall cost of early intervention with chemotherapy in patients with advanced colorectal cancer is similar to that of no treatment or delayed chemotherapy, indicating that chemotherapy as part of the management of the advanced disease is indeed cost effective. Inevitably, it is becoming increasingly difficult for the health service to fund modern drugs to treat advanced colorectal cancer. The NHS is struggling to fund the new chemotherapy treatments that are proved to extend life by only a few months or to improve the quality of life only.

Ambulatory and domiciliary chemotherapy

The emergence of primary care health teams, together with developing technology, has allowed for more complex care to be carried out in the community or at home.

Ambulatory infusional chemotherapy is administered via a small pump (battery assisted and disposable elastomeric infuser). The chemotherapy may be connected and disconnected at the hospital outpatient clinic by oncology nurses, or patients can be taught to do this themselves.

A feasibility study of home chemotherapy has been undertaken in Birmingham for patients with advanced colorectal cancer. This shows that a nurse led service (backed up by oncology medical and nursing staff from both primary and secondary health care) is safe and that patients and carers find home therapy of immeasurable value. Early analysis shows that the cost of this home service is similar to and often cheaper than the current hospital based service.

New drugs

In recent years the availability of several new drugs has revived interest in the treatment of advanced colorectal cancer. New treatments include alternative fluoropyrimidines, new thymidylate synthase inhibitors, new modulators of fluorouracil and also mechanistically new drugs.

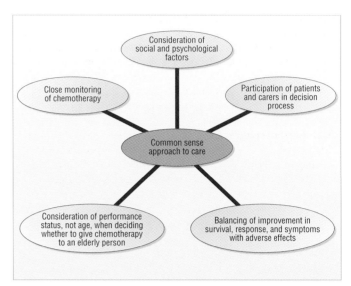

Figure 8.2 Basic elements of caring for patients with advanced colorectal cancer

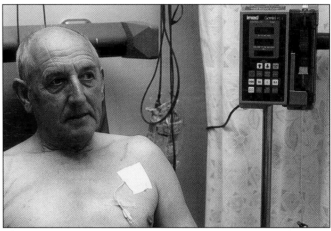

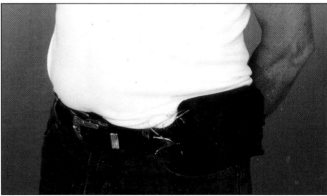

Figure 8.3 Patient receiving chemotherapy through central venous catheter in hospital outpatient department (top); and small, battery assisted pump, worn on the waist and used to deliver chemotherapy through a central venous catheter (bottom). Patients are free to perform many normal activities during "ambulatory" chemotherapy

---

Box 8.5 Current controversies in advanced colorectal cancer

- For how long should chemotherapy be given?
- Are new delivery routes for fluorouracil—for example, orally and by intrahepatic arterial administration—superior to conventional intravenous fluorouracil?
- Should newer agents with similar efficacy but more convenient intravenous regimens be used in place of fluorouracil?
- What is the optimum combination and sequence for fluorouracil based therapies and the new chemotherapy drugs?
- Is home chemotherapy viable?
- How are the new, more expensive drug therapies to be funded?

New thymidylate synthase inhibitors

Raltitrexed is a quinazoline analogue antifolate that gains entry to cells via the reduced folate carrier and is polyglutamated to a potent, long acting, specific inhibitor of thymidylate synthase. Its regimen—a short intravenous infusion every three weeks—has similar efficacy to that of fluorouracil plus folinic acid and is clearly more convenient, although potentially more toxic.

Oral fluorouracil prodrugs and modulators

Fluoropyrimidine analogues have been developed with reliable oral bioavailability. In addition, oral inhibitors of fluorouracil catabolism can facilitate oral dosing. Preliminary data show similar effectiveness and lower toxicity compared with fluorouracil. Given the convenience and potential cost savings, oral therapy may soon find a place in routine practice.

Irinotecan and oxaliplatin

Irinotecan is a camptothecin analogue that acts through the inhibition of a DNA unwinding enzyme, topoisomerase I, resulting in replication arrest with breaks in single strand DNA. It is useful in advanced colorectal cancer, even after resistance to fluorouracil has developed, and is associated with a survival benefit (about three months) compared with best supportive care. This drug can be associated with severe late onset diarrhoea, which must be treated immediately. Selection of patients, therefore, plays an important part in the safe use of this agent.

Oxaliplatin is a new platinum derivative analogue that crosslinks DNA and induces apoptotic cell death. It shows synergism with fluorouracil. The dominant toxic effect is cumulative neurotoxicity.

Fluorouracil plus either irinotecan or oxaliplatin is superior to fluorouracil alone as a first line treatment for advanced colorectal cancer, with improvement in progression-free survival and, in the case of irinotecan, overall survival. Questions about the optimum sequence and combination of these agents remain and are the subject of ongoing clinical trials.

Intrahepatic arterial chemotherapy

For patients with unresectable hepatic metastases, intrahepatic arterial chemotherapy should be considered. This approach greatly increases drug delivery to the liver and doubles the rate at which tumours shrink, with tolerable toxicity. Owing to the complexity of placing the delivery catheter, intrahepatic arterial chemotherapy is usually administered at specialist centres. Current trials should offer definitive proof of whether intrahepatic arterial chemotherapy offers survival benefits compared with conventional intravenous therapy.

Supportive care

All patients with advanced colorectal cancer need continual evaluation of symptoms and appropriate measures for controlling symptoms. Dietary advice and nutritional supplements can stop weight loss, and corticosteroids may be used for their anabolic effect. Psychosocial aspects of care should incorporate evaluation of and provision for the needs of both the patient and the family. Supportive care needs to be tailored to the individual's circumstances and should involve the close collaboration of locally available palliative care services (both in the community and in hospitals). The initial contact between the patient and the palliative team should ideally be made at the time of diagnosis rather than at a crisis point when urgent input from palliative care services is required.

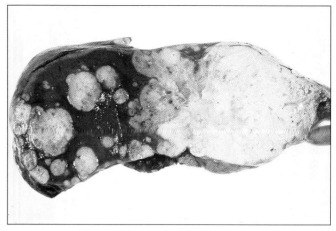

Figure 8.4 Liver with over 50% hepatic replacement by metastatic colorectal cancer

The Colorectal Forum is a worldwide educational service for healthcare professionals working with patients with colorectal cancer. Its website provides news on conferences and events, recommendations on management of advanced colorectal cancer, articles and visual images, reviews of recent publications, and the opportunity to debate controversial clinical issues. It can be accessed at www.colorectal-forum.org

Further reading

- *A policy framework for commissioning cancer services*. London: Department of Health, 1994. (Consultative document.)
- Clinical Outcomes Group. *Guidance on commissioning cancer services: improving outcomes in colorectal cancer*. London: NHS Executive, 1997.
- Cady B, Stone M. The role of surgical resection of liver metastases in colorectal carcinoma. *Semin Oncol* 1991;18:399-406.
- Nordic Gastrointestinal Tumour Adjuvant Therapy Group. Expectancy or primary chemotherapy in patients with advanced, asymptomatic colorectal cancer: a randomised trial. *J Clin Oncol* 1992;10:904-11.
- Glimelius B, Hoffman K, Graf W, Haglund U, Nyren O, Pahlman L, et al. Cost-effectiveness of palliative chemotherapy in advanced gastrointestinal cancer. *Ann Oncol* 1995;6:267-74.

9 Effectiveness of follow up

Colin McArdle

Population based studies show that for rectal cancer the incidence of local recurrence after apparently curative resection is about 20%. Local recurrence after surgery for colon cancer is less common. The liver is the commonest site of distant spread, followed by the lungs; brain and bone metastases are relatively rare. Most recurrences are within 24 months of surgery.

Aim of follow up

Traditionally surgeons have reviewed their patients at regular intervals after apparently curative resection. Recent surveys, however, have highlighted the lack of consensus among surgeons about the optimal modality and intensity of follow up; surveillance strategies range from a single postoperative visit to lifelong surveillance. Enthusiasts believe that intensive follow up and early intervention will lead to a reduction in the number of deaths from colorectal cancer; others point to the fact that the value of follow up is unproved. With so many tests available and no consensus on their value, it is not surprising that individual clinicians have tended to devise their own protocols.

Box 9.1 Aims of follow up
- Early detection and treatment of recurrent disease
- Detection of a second, or metachronous, tumour in the large bowel
- Provision of psychological support and advice
- Facilitation of audit

Results of meta-analysis

A meta-analysis in the mid-1990s did little to clarify the situation. The researchers evaluated the results of seven non-randomised studies (covering over 3000 subjects in total) that compared intensive follow up with minimal or no follow up. Clearly several potential biases could and did exist. In the intensive group, investigations included clinical examination, faecal occult blood testing, liver function tests, measurement of the carcinoembyronic antigen, sigmoidoscopy, and either colonoscopy or barium enema examination. Liver ultrasonography was performed in only three studies and even then infrequently. In the intensive group more asymptomatic recurrences were detected, more patients underwent "second look" laparotomy, and more patients had a second potentially curative resection; more metachronous tumours were also detected and resected. However, although there were fewer deaths in the group receiving intensive follow up, this difference did not reach significance.

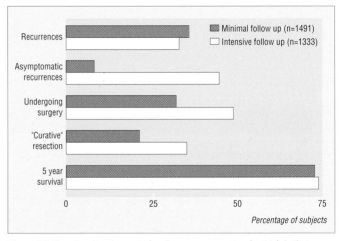

Figure 9.1 Results of meta-analysis of seven non-randomised trials that compared intensive with minimal or no follow up (Bruinvels et al, 1994)

Results of randomised clinical trials

Since the meta-analysis, four randomised trials of intensive follow up have been reported. Ohlsson and his colleagues randomised 107 patients to no follow up or to intensive follow up, similar to that described above. No liver imaging was performed routinely. No differences were found in recurrence rates or in overall or cancer specific mortality.

Mákelá and his associates compared conventional with intensive follow up in 106 patients. In the intensive group flexible sigmoidoscopy was performed every three months, ultrasonography every six months, and colonoscopy and abdominal computed tomography at yearly intervals. Recurrences were detected at an earlier stage (median 10 months v 15 months) in the intensive group. Despite this, no difference in survival was found between the two groups.

Kjeldsen and his colleagues randomised almost 600 patients to either six monthly follow up or to follow up visits at five and 10 years only. Investigations included chest x ray and colonoscopy; no routine liver imaging was performed. Recurrence rates were similar (26%) in both groups, but the recurrences in the intensive group were detected on average nine months earlier, often at an asymptomatic stage. More patients with local recurrence underwent repeat surgery with curative intent. No difference existed, however, in overall survival (68% v 70%) or cancer related survival.

More recently, Schoemaker and his colleagues evaluated the addition of annual chest radiography, colonoscopy, and computed tomography of the liver to a standard follow up based on clinical examination, faecal occult blood testing, liver function tests, and measurement of the carcinoembyronic antigen, with further investigations as clinically indicated. At five years, fewer patients in the intensive group had died, but the result was not significant. At the cost of 505 additional investigations, annual colonoscopy failed to detect any asymptomatic local recurrences; only one asymptomatic metachronous colon tumour was detected. Six hundred and eight additional liver computed tomograms detected only one asymptomatic patient with liver metastases who might have benefited from liver resection.

Carcinoembryonic antigen

Carcinoembryonic antigen concentrations have also been used to predict recurrence. About three quarters of patients with recurrent colorectal cancer have a raised carcinoembryonic antigen concentration before developing symptoms.

An alternative approach therefore would be to monitor this concentration regularly during follow up and, in those patients showing a rising concentration, undertake second look laparotomy. However, although early non-randomised studies suggested that surgery that was prompted by this method resulted in more potentially curative repeat operations for recurrence, more recent studies have failed to show a survival advantage.

Moertel analysed outcome in patients included in trials of adjuvant therapy, according to whether the patient underwent carcinoembryonic antigen testing. Of 1017 patients whose concentrations were monitored, 417 (41%) developed recurrence. A comparison of those patients whose follow up included measurements of carcinoembryonic antigen with those whose follow up did not, failed to show any difference in disease-free survival. Among 29 laparotomies performed solely on the basis of a raised concentration of carcinoembryonic antigen, only one patient remained alive and disease-free after one year.

In the randomised study by Northover and his colleagues, 1447 patients undergoing potentially curative surgery were randomised to an intervention group or a control group. Carcinoembryonic antigen was measured in all patients at frequent intervals. In the intervention group, a rising antigen concentration prompted further investigation, including second look laparotomy, if appropriate.

Preliminary analysis showed no difference in survival between the two groups. The failure to show a survival advantage in the intervention group may be due to the fact that a rising antigen concentration is a relatively poor predictor of local recurrence; furthermore, even in patients with liver metastases a rising concentration is a relatively late phenomenon.

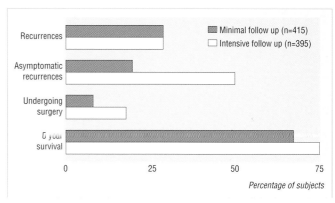

Figure 9.2 Combined results of three randomised trials of intensive follow up

Table 9.1 Results of intensive follow up*

Follow up	Colonoscopy	Chest x ray	Liver CT
Standard (n = 158)	72	17	66
Intensive (n = 167)	577	650	674
No of extra investigations	505	633	608
No of asymptomatic recurrences resulting from extra investigations	0	0	10
No of cures resulting from extra investigations	0	1	1

CT = computed tomography.
*Data from Schoemaker et al, 1998 (see Further reading box).

> **Carcinoembryonic antigen concentrations have been used to predict recurrence of colorectal cancer, but recent evidence does not support this approach**

Table 9.2 Results of "second look" surgery according to measurement of carcinoembryonic antigen (CEA)*

CEA concentration	No of patients	No (%) of "curative" resections	% of patients free of recurrence at 1 year
Raised	345	47 (14)	2.9
Normal	672	38 (6)	1.9
Not measured	200	23 (12)	2.0

*Data from Moertel et al, 1993.

31

Cost effectiveness

Concern is also increasing about the cost of follow up. A review of the published literature suggests a 28-fold difference in costs between the least intensive and most intensive, published, five year follow up protocols.

Wrong target?

Clearly, follow up as currently practised is ineffective. Why, therefore, should we continue to follow patients up after apparently curative resection for colorectal cancer? There are several reasons. Firstly, we should do so to provide psychological support and advice; many patients welcome the reassurance that regular check up provides. Secondly, routine follow up facilitates audit of outcome measures after surgery, ensures quality control and facilitates evaluation of trials of new treatments and strategies.

There may, however, be a more fundamental reason that current follow up practices are ineffective. On theoretical grounds, attempts to identify potentially resectable local recurrences or metachronous tumours were never likely to have a significant impact on survival. Isolated resectable anastomotic recurrences are uncommon. Most local recurrences arise from residual disease left at the time of surgery and therefore, by definition, are unlikely to be amenable to further curative surgery. Metachronous tumours, although potentially amenable to surgery, are relatively uncommon.

Wrong intervention?

In contrast, liver metastases are much more common. Furthermore, these metastases are confined to the liver in about a quarter of patients.

Perhaps, therefore, the emphasis should shift towards the early detection of liver metastases. It is worth noting that in contemporary studies of liver resection, mortality is less than 5% and about 35% of patients survive five years. These figures are better than the results obtained after primary surgery for many types of gastrointestinal cancer. Furthermore recent studies have shown that patients with disseminated disease who receive systemic chemotherapy at an asymptomatic stage have higher response rates, better quality of life, and improved survival compared with those in whom the administration of chemotherapy is delayed until symptoms appear. Therefore if liver metastases were diagnosed in more patients at a point at which they were amenable to resection or chemotherapy, more long term survivors might be anticipated.

To date only two randomised studies have included liver imaging. In both these studies the numbers were small and liver imaging was infrequent. In neither study was a survival advantage noted. However, intensive liver imaging for the first three years after surgery may be more effective: at the Royal Infirmary in Glasgow more than 80% of patients who developed liver metastases as the initial site of recurrence were detected at an asymptomatic stage.

Hospital or community coordination of follow up?

Most patients with colorectal cancer are followed up in hospital. Yet overwhelming evidence from previous studies shows that few curable recurrences are detected at routine follow up based on history, physical examination, and routine blood tests. Few patients are followed up by their general practitioners, although

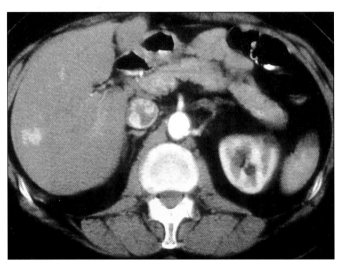

Figure 9.3 Contrast enhanced computed tomogram (arterial phase) showing solitary liver metastasis

Table 9.3 Comparison of results of trial of early versus delayed chemotherapy in patients with advanced colorectal cancer

Treatment group	No of patients	Median symptom-free survival (months)	Median survival (months)	Survival at 1 year (%)
Early	92	10	14	55
Delayed	91	2	9	38

Early chemotherapy was given when patients were asymptomatic; delayed chemotherapy was given when patients were symptomatic.
Data from the Nordic Gastrointestinal Tumor Group, 1992.

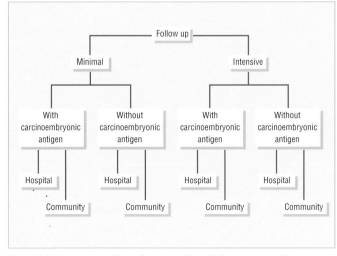

Figure 9.4 Suggested study outline to test three follow up strategies: intensive *v* minimalist; role of carcinoembyronic antigen; and general practitioner (community) coordinated *v* hospital coordinated

good evidence exists that, in other tumours at least, such follow up is as effective (or ineffective) as hospital follow up. Furthermore, provided that general practitioners have access to a "fast track" referral system for patients in whom they suspected recurrent disease, follow up coordinated by general practitioners might offer several advantages. It might be more acceptable to and convenient for patients and might reduce costs.

Perhaps it is time to reassess follow up. Formal studies to assess the value of these strategies might include:
● A comparison of the value of intensive versus minimalist follow up
● A re-evaluation of the role of carcinoembyronic antigen
● A comparison of the effectiveness of follow up that is coordinated by general practitioners rather than by hospitals.

Conclusion

Current methods of follow up, aimed at the early detection and treatment of local recurrence or metachronous tumours, have yet to be shown to be cost effective.

As liver metastases are common, a protocol that includes regular liver imaging to detect potentially resectable lesions may prove more effective. Further studies are needed to assess the value of this approach in patients undergoing apparently curative resection for colorectal cancer.

Further reading

● Bruinvels DJ, Stiggelbout AM, Kievit J, Van Houwelingen HC, Habbema JDF, van de Velde CJH. Follow-up of patients with colorectal cancer: a meta-analysis. *Ann Surg* 1994;219:174-82.
● Kjeldsen B, Kronberg O, Fenger C, Jorgensen O. A prospective randomised study of follow-up after radical surgery for colorectal cancer. *Br J Surg* 1997;84:666-9.
● Mákelá JT, Laitinen SO, Kairaluoma MI. Five year follow-up after radical surgery for colorectal cancer: results of a prospective randomised trial. *Arch Surg* 1995;130:1062-7.
● Ohlsson B, Breland U, Ekberg H, Graffner H, Tranberg K. Follow-up after curative surgery for colorectal carcinoma: randomised comparison with no follow-up. *Dis Colon Rectum* 1995;38:619-26.
● Schoemaker D, Black R, Giles L, Toouli J. Yearly colonoscopy, liver CT, and chest radiography do not influence 5-year survival of colorectal cancer patients. *Gastroenterology* 1998;114:7-14.

10 Innovative treatment for colon cancer

G A Chung-Faye, D J Kerr

Despite advances in treatment for colon cancer, the five year survival has not significantly altered over the past decade. Survival could improve in several key areas:
- Preventive measures—such as diet and chemoprevention with agents such as non-steroidal anti-inflammatory drugs
- Screening strategies—such as faecal occult blood testing and flexible sigmoidoscopy
- Optimisation of current chemotherapy and radiotherapy regimens and the development of more effective antineoplastic agents
- New therapeutic approaches—such as immunotherapy and gene therapy.

This article will focus on prevention with non-steroidal anti-inflammatory drugs and on new strategies for treating colon cancer.

Non-steroidal anti-inflammatory drugs

Evidence strongly suggests a protective effect of non-steroidal anti-inflammatory drugs in colon cancer. Several cohort and case-control studies have consistently shown dose related reductions of colorectal cancer in regular users of these drugs. Furthermore, patients with familial adenomatous polyposis who took the non-steroidal anti-inflammatory sulindac had reductions in the number and size of their polyps. Gene knockout studies in mice suggest that inhibition of the cyclo-oxygenase type 2 pathway by non-steroidal anti-inflammatory drugs may be important in the mechanism of action.

The only randomised controlled trial examining the effect of aspirin in primary prevention of colon cancer did not show any benefit after five years of aspirin use. A recent prospective cohort study suggested, however, that five years may be insufficient to show any benefit and that 10-20 years is needed to show an effect.

The predominant side effect from using non-steroidal anti-inflammatory drugs is the increased incidence of gastrointestinal bleeds. On the current evidence, the mortality risk from such bleeding would be outweighed by the reduction in mortality from colon cancer. To maximise the benefit to risk ratio, however, targeting individuals at high risk of colon cancer may prove more fruitful.

Non-steroidal anti-inflammatory drugs could be used as secondary prevention after surgical resection of colonic tumours, but this approach has yet to be tested in a large randomised controlled trial.

Immunotherapy

Many cancers can be destroyed by a tumour specific, cell mediated immune response, usually by CD8 (cytotoxic) lymphocytes. However, colorectal tumours are poorly immunogenic and may evade immune destruction by various mechanisms, such as tumour "tolerance." To overcome these problems, several immunostimulatory approaches have been advocated to augment the innate immune response against tumours.

Dietary modifications to reduce the incidence of colon cancer may be difficult to implement (dietary interventional studies have shown this to be the case for cardiovascular disease); the roles of screening, chemotherapy, and radiotherapy have been covered earlier in this series

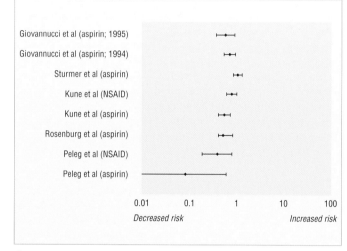

Figure 10.1 Use of non-steroidal anti-inflammatory drugs (NSAID) and relative risk of colorectal cancer

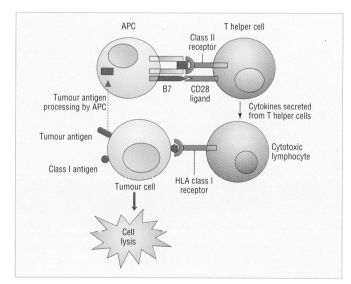

Figure 10.2 Cell mediated immunity against tumours. Tumour antigens are taken up and processed by antigen presenting cells (APC) and re-presented to class II receptors on T helper cells. This requires a costimulatory signal, B7, which binds to the CD28 ligand, causing T helper cell activation. This leads to secretion of cytokines, which in turn activates cytotoxic lymphocytes to bind to tumour cells via class I receptors and causes tumour lysis

Vaccination with autologous tumour cells

This approach uses cells derived from the patient's tumour to elicit a cell mediated immune response against the tumour. To increase the efficacy of this response, tumour cells are coadministered with an immunomodulatory adjuvant, such as BCG. This approach has been tested in three randomised, controlled trials in an adjuvant setting in colorectal cancer, after resection of the tumour. No serious side effects were encountered in any of the studies.

Vaccination against tumour associated antigens

An alternative approach is vaccination against a tumour associated antigen, such as the carcinoembryonic antigen, which is overexpressed in 90% of colon cancers. A phase I immunisation study of a recombinant vaccinia virus, encoding the gene for carcinoembryonic antigen, in patients with advanced colorectal cancer, showed HLA specific, cytolytic T cell responses to carcinoembryonic antigen epitopes in vitro. This study did not show any clinical benefit, but several trials are under way, using optimal vaccination approaches in patients with minimal residual disease where clinical responses may be observed.

Monoclonal antibodies directed against tumour antigens

Monoclonal antibodies against tumour antigens have been shown to elicit immune responses against the tumour, which may previously have induced immunogenic tolerance. The 17-1A antigen is a surface glycoprotein with a putative role in cell adhesion and is present in over 90% of colorectal tumours.

In a study among patients with Dukes's stage C colon cancer the patients were randomised to receive either surgery alone or surgery plus repeat administrations of a monoclonal antibody against the 17-1A antigen. Side effects of the treatment were infrequent, consisting mainly of mild constitutional and gastrointestinal symptoms. Four patients experienced an anaphylactic reaction, which required intravenous steroids but no hospital admission.

Gene therapy

Gene therapy represents a new treatment approach for colon cancer. It is at a developmental stage, and preclinical studies are only just being translated into clinical trials. Two gene therapy strategies are currently used, gene correction and enzyme-prodrug systems.

Gene correction

The most logical approach to gene therapy is the correction of a single gene defect, which causes the disease phenotype. In colon cancer, as in many other cancers, this goal is elusive as malignant transformation is usually accompanied by a series of genetic mutations. However, some of these mutations, such as the p53 gene mutation, are important for the propagation of the malignant phenotype, and the corollary is that correcting these mutations may inhibit the growth of tumour cells.

P53 gene

The p53 gene regulates the cell cycle and can cause growth arrest or apoptosis in response to DNA damage. Loss of p53 control leads to uncontrolled growth and is associated with more aggressive tumours. Restoration of wild-type p53 in p53 mutated tumours inhibits growth. In a phase I trial an adenovirus encoding wild-type p53 was delivered by hepatic artery infusion to 16 patients with p53 mutated colorectal liver metastases. This procedure was well tolerated, with the side

---

Box 10.1 Immunostimulatory approaches for augmenting the innate immune response against tumours

- Vaccination with autologous tumour cells
- Vaccination against tumour associated antigens, such as carcinoembryonic antigen
- Use of monoclonal antibodies directed against tumour antigens

---

Box 10.2 Vaccination with autologous tumour cells

Hoover et al, 1993
- 98 patients with colon or rectal cancer were randomised to surgery alone or to surgery plus vaccination with autologous tumour cells
- No significant improvement in the recurrence or the survival rate
- Subgroup analysis of patients with colon cancer showed a significant improvement in survival and disease-free survival in those who received vaccination (P = 0.02, P = 0.039 respectively)

Harris et al, 1994
- 412 patients with Dukes's stage B and C colon cancer were postoperatively randomised to vaccination with autologous tumour cells or to no further treatment
- No significant differences between treated and untreated groups

Vermorken et al, 1999
- 254 postoperative patients with stage II or III colon cancer were randomised to vaccination with autologous tumour cells or to no further treatment. Those randomised to receive vaccination received a 4th booster vaccine after six months (in contrast with the patients in the two previous studies, who received only three doses)
- In the those receiving vaccination, there was a significant reduction in recurrence (44%, 95% confidence interval 7% to 66%) and a reduction in overall survival, although this did not reach significance
- The main benefit was in stage II disease, with a non-significant reduction in recurrence in stage III disease; this was thought to be due to the increased tumour burden in more advanced stages

---

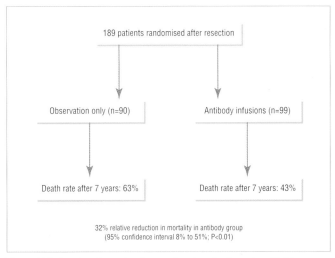

Figure 10.3 Results of a study of monoclonal antibody against 17-1A as adjuvant therapy in Dukes's C colon cancer (Riethmuller et al, 1998)

The p53 gene mutation is present in most colon cancers

effects of fever and transiently damaged liver function. Although gene expression was detected in subsequently resected tumours, no radiographic responses were seen at 28 days. This study has now proceeded to a phase II trial, in combination with intrahepatic floxuridine based chemotherapy, in which 11 out of 12 patients have had partial responses.

Virus directed enzyme-prodrug treatment

Enzyme-prodrug systems are used to localise the toxic drug effects to tumour cells. This involves gene transfer of an enzyme into tumour cells, which converts an inactive prodrug into a toxic metabolite, leading to cell death. An important feature of enzyme-prodrug systems is the "bystander effect," whereby surrounding cells (not expressing the enzyme) are also killed by active metabolites. Gene transfer is achieved by viral vectors, such as retroviruses or adenoviruses. One such enzyme-prodrug combination is the bacterial enzyme cytosine deaminase, which converts the antifungal agent fluorocytosine into the antineoplastic agent fluorouracil. Fluorouracil induces apoptosis by inhibition of the enzyme thymidylate synthase during DNA replication. In murine models with colon cancer xenografts expressing cytosine deaminase, 75% of mice were cured by administration of fluorocytosine, whereas no anti-tumour effect was seen with the maximally tolerated dose of fluorouracil.

New therapeutic agents

The matrix metalloproteinases are a group of enzymes involved in the physiological maintenance of the extracellular matrix. They degrade the extracellular matrix and promote the formation of new blood vessels and are involved in tissue remodelling processes, such as wound healing and angiogenesis. Matrix metalloproteinases are overexpressed, however, in various tumours, including colorectal cancers, and have been implicated in facilitating tumour invasion and metastasis. The matrix metalloproteinase inhibitor, marimastat, has shown reductions in levels of tumour markers in phase I studies, and its clinical efficacy is currently being tested in phase III trials.

Conclusions

Non-steroidal anti-inflammatory drugs seem to be the most promising drug for prevention of colon cancer; case-control and prospective cohort studies strongly suggest they reduce the risk of colon cancer. This is further supported by studies in familial cancer patients and animal data. However, this effect of non-steroidal anti-inflammatory drugs is unproved in randomised controlled trials, and the issue remains to be addressed.

Immunotherapy seems to be well tolerated and effective in an adjuvant setting in colon cancer with limited residual disease. Its effect in stage II disease is comparable to that of adjuvant chemotherapy in Dukes's C colon cancer. In more advanced disease it may have a role in combination with chemotherapy, and this approach is being explored in ongoing trials.

Gene therapy for colon cancer is still at an early stage of development. Preclinical studies have prompted several phase I trials. However, significant problems remain, such as low efficiency in gene transfer and the inhibitory effect of the host immunity, which may be addressed by developments in vector technology. As our understanding of the molecular biology of cancer increases, gene therapy is likely to have an increasingly important role in the expanding array of treatment options for colon cancer.

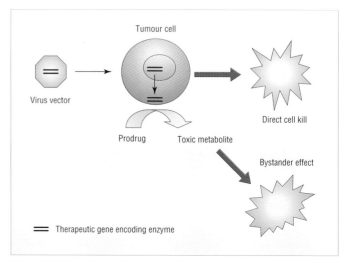

Figure 10.4 Virus directed enzyme-prodrug treatment

Two current phase I trials are using a virus directed enzyme-prodrugs approach for treating colorectal liver metastases by direct injection into the tumour of an adenovirus encoding a therapeutic enzyme. One study is using nitroreductase plus the intravenous prodrug CB1954; the other is using cytosine deaminase plus fluorocytosine

Further reading

- Langman M, Boyle P. Chemoprevention of colorectal cancer. *Gut* 1998;43:578-85.
- Gann PH, Manson JE, Glynn RJ, Buring JE, Hennekens CH. Low-dose aspirin and incidence of colorectal tumors in a randomized trial. *J Natl Cancer Institute* 1993;85:1220-4.
- Vermorken JB, Claessen AME, van Tintern H, Gall HE, Ezinga R, Meijer S, et al. Active specific immunotherapy for stage II and stage III human colon cancer: a randomised trial. *Lancet* 1999;353:345-50.
- Riethmuller G, Holz E, Schlimok G, Schmiegel W, Raab R, Hoffken K, et al. Monoclonal antibody therapy for resected Dukes' C colorectal cancer: seven-year outcome of a multicenter randomized trial. *J Clin Oncol* 1998;16:1788-94.
- Roth JA, Cristiano RJ. Gene therapy for cancer: what have we done and where are we going? *J Natl Cancer Institute* 1997;89:21-39.
- Chung-Faye GA, Kerr DJ, Young LS, Searle PF. Gene therapy strategies for colon cancer. *Molecular Medicine Today* 2000;6:82-7.

Index